A Nurse's Handbook of Spiritual Care:

STANDING ON HOLY GROUND

MARY ELIZABETH O'BRIEN, SFCC
PHD, MTS, RN, FAAN

*The Catholic University of America
School of Nursing*

JONES AND BARTLETT PUBLISHERS
Sudbury, Massachusetts
BOSTON   TORONTO   LONDON   SINGAPORE

World Headquarters

Jones and Bartlett Publishers
40 Tall Pine Drive
Sudbury, MA 01776
978-443-5000
info@jbpub.com
www.jbpub.com

Jones and Bartlett Publishers Canada
2406 Nikanna Road
Mississauga, ON L5C 2W6
CANADA

Jones and Bartlett Publishers International
Barb House, Barb Mews
London W6 7PA
UK

Library of Congress Cataloging-in-Publication Data not available at time of printing.

ISBN: 0-7637-3291-5

Production Credits

Acquisitions Editor: Kevin Sullivan
Production Manager: Amy Rose
Associate Production Editor: Karen C. Ferreira
Editorial Assistant: Amy Sibley
Associate Marketing Manager: Joy Stark-Vancs
Marketing Associate: Elizabeth Waterfall
Manufacturing and Inventory Coordinator: Amy Bacus
Cover Design: Kristin E. Ohlin
Composition: AnnMarie Lemoine
Printing and Binding: United Graphics Incorporated
Cover Printing: United Graphics Incorporated

Printed in the United States of America
07 06 05 04 03   10 9 8 7 6 5 4 3 2 1

A Nurse's Handbook of Spiritual Care
is lovingly dedicated to all nurses who
"stand on holy ground" in their blessed
ministry of caring and compassion.

God called (to Moses) out of the bush: . . . "Remove the sandals from your feet, for the place on which you are standing is holy ground."

Exodus 3:4–5

The nurse's smile warmly embraces the cancer patient arriving for a chemotherapy treatment.
    This is holy ground.
The nurse watches solicitously over the pre-op child who tearfully whispers "I'm scared."
    This is holy ground.
The nurse gently diffuses the anxieties of the ventilator-dependent patient in the ICU.
    This is holy ground.
The nurse lovingly sings hymns to the anencephalic infant dying in the nurse's arms.
    This is holy ground.
The nurse slips a comforting arm around the trembling shoulders of the newly bereaved widow.
    This is holy ground.
The nurse tenderly takes the hand of the frail elder struggling to accept life in the nursing home.
    This is holy ground.
The nurse reverently touches and is touched by the patient's heart, the dwelling place of the living God.
    This is spirituality in nursing,
    this is the ground of the practice of nursing,
    this is holy ground!

Preface

A Nurse's Handbook of Spiritual Care contains material previously found in *Spirituality In Nursing: Standing On Holy Ground*. Major portions of that text are included, especially such topics as: the nurse's role in spiritual care; the assessment of patients' spiritual needs; nursing diagnoses related to alterations in spiritual integrity; the nurse-patient covenant; spiritual needs of the acutely ill person; spiritual needs of the chronically ill person; spiritual needs of children and families; spiritual needs of the older adult; spiritual needs in death and bereavement; spiritual needs in mass casualty trauma; and parish nursing.

The *Handbook* also contains numerous meditations and prayers for nurses taken from *Prayer In Nursing: The Spirituality of Compassionate Caregiveing* and *Parish Nursing: Healthcare Ministry within the Church*. Fifteen "Nurses' Prayers For the Sick" are included, focusing on such patient needs as: "Prayer for a Person Preparing to Enter the Hospital," "Prayer Before Surgery," "Prayer for a Sick Child," "Prayer for a Person Beginning Life in a Nursing Home," "Prayer for One Who is Terminally Ill," "Prayer for Discontinuing Life Support."

Additionally, the *Handbook* contains a spiritual assessment tool and a model that nurses may find useful in clinical practice or research: the "Spiritual Assessment Scale" and the "Model of Spiritual Well-Being in Illness." A revised chapter on parish nursing includes a "Parish Health Needs Assessment" form and six tables that describe: "Guidelines for Developing a Parish Health Ministry Program"; "Suggested Activities for Parish Health Ministers"; "Ministry Visits to Homebound Parishioners";

"Ministry Visits to Hospitalized Parishioners"; "Ministry Visits to Parishioners in Long-term Care Facilities"; and "Ministry Visits to Terminally Ill Parishioners" and "Bereaved Families."

A final chapter on "Prayer in Nursing: the Spirituality of Compassionate Caregiving" summarizes major elements from the book *Prayer in Nursing*, such as a history of prayer in nursing, praying with scripture, finding time for prayer in nursing, and steps to facilitate a time of prayer.

The combining, in this *Nurse's Handbook of Spiritual Care*, of key portions of text, references, meditations, prayers, assessment tools, and guidelines for spiritual care from three earlier books will facilitate use of the material for nurses practicing in myriad settings such as hospitals, hospices, nursing homes, assisted care facilities, clinics, physician's offices, homes and parishes.

Acknowledgments ─────────

The words to acknowledge all of the people involved in creating a book are never adequate; as I have written before, "it takes a village." I have already thanked, and continue to deeply appreciate, the many colleagues and friends who taught, encouraged and supported the writing of *Spirituality in Nursing: Standing On Holy Ground*, *Prayer In Nursing: The Spirituality of Compassionate Caregiving*, and *Parish Nursing: Healthcare Ministry within the Church*.

For the birthing of this, *A Nurses' Handbook of Spiritual Care*, however, I want especially to acknowledge the editorial staff of Jones and Bartlett Publishers: Joy Stark-Vancs, who conceived the idea of a "handbook"; Kevin Sullivan, who convinced me that the book could be a useful guide for nurses; and Karen Ferreira, who advised on organization of the content.

Finally, as always, my greatest gratitude is to God, the Father, to His Son, Our Lord Jesus Christ, and to the Holy Spirit of Wisdom and Understanding; they are the true authors of this work. The Lord is the master musician; I am simply His small flute.

Contents

Note: 🔥 indicates a prayer.

8   Spiritual Care of the Older Adult   103

9   Spiritual Care in Death and Bereavement   117

Epilogue 181

Appendix A: Nurses' Prayers 183
for the Sick

Appendix B: A Nurse's Psalm of Reverence for Life

Appendix C: A Nurse's Way of the Cross

Index

Scripture Index

Also by Mary Elizabeth O'Brien

Parish Nursing: Healthcare Ministry within the Church

Prayer in Nursing: The Art of Compassionate Caregiving

Spirituality in Nursing: Standing on Holy Ground, Second Edition

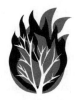

CHAPTER 1

Spirituality in Nursing: Standing on Holy Ground

Remove the sandals from your feet, for the place on which you are standing is holy ground.

EXODUS 3:5

Remove the Sandals from Your Feet

Lord God of Israel,
You taught us, through Moses,
that when we stand before You,
the ground is holy and we must
"remove the sandals from our feet" (Exodus 3:5)

But. . .
removing the sandals from our feet may leave us:
anxious,
vulnerable,
fragile,
insecure,
penitent,
and yet receptive; and humbly open to Your compassion and Your care.

Teach us to "remove the sandals from our feet"
permanently, that we may stand forever on the "holy ground" of Your Blessed Presence.

Perhaps no scriptural theme so well models the spiritual posture of nursing practice as the Old Testament depiction of Moses and the burning bush. In the biblical narrative, God reminded Moses that, when he stood before his Lord, the ground beneath his feet was holy. When the nurse clinician, nurse educator, nurse administrator, or nurse researcher stands before a patient, a student, a staff member, or a study participant, God is also present, and the ground on which the nurse is standing is holy. For it is here, in the act of serving a brother or sister in need, that the nurse truly encounters God. God is present in the nurse's practice of caring just as surely as He was present in the blessed meeting with Moses so many centuries ago.

The Nurse's Role is Spiritual Care: Standing on Holy Ground

Nursing may be described as a sacred ministry of health care or health promotion provided to persons both sick and well, who require caregiving, support, or education to assist them in achieving, regaining, or maintaining a state of wholeness, including wellness of body, mind, and spirit. The nurse also serves those in need of comfort and care to strengthen them in coping with the trajectory of a chronic or terminal illness, or with experiencing the dying process.

The spiritual dimensions of the definition encompass two concepts: first, the sacred ministry of caring on the part of the nurse; and second, the ultimate goal of the patient's achievement of a state of wholeness, including the wellness of body, mind, and spirit. Spiritual writer Macrina Wiederkehr (1991) advised: "If you should ever hear God speaking to you from a burning bush, and it happens more often than most of us realize, take off your shoes for the ground on which you stand is holy" (p. 2). How appropriate, it seems, to envision practicing nurses, who must come together with their patients in caring and compassion, as standing on holy ground. God frequently speaks to us from a "burning bush," in the fretful whimper of a feverish child, in the anxious questions of a preoperative surgical patient, and in the frail moans of a fragile elder. If we "take off our shoes," we will be able to realize that the place where we stand is holy ground; we will respond to our patients as we would wish to respond to God in the burning bush.

Holistic Nursing: The Body, Mind, and Spirit Connection

At times one hears an individual described as being truly healthy. The assumption underlying such a remark may relate not so much to the physical health or well-being of the person as to the fact that he or she is perceived as solidly grounded spiritually. One can be possessed of a healthy attitude toward life, even if suffering from a terminal illness. In order to achieve such a spiritual grounding in the face of physical or psychological deficit, the individual must be closely attuned to the body, mind, and spirit connection; one must understand and accept the value of the spiritual dimension in the overall paradigm of holistic health.

Holistic nursing is supported by and alternately supports this intimate connection of body, mind, and spirit. Nursing of the whole person requires attention to the individuality and uniqueness of each dimension, as well as to the interrelatedness of the three. For the nurse seeking to provide holistic health care, then, the spiritual dimension and needs of the person must be carefully assessed and considered in all therapeutic planning. Spiritual care cannot be separated from physical, social, and psychological care. Often it is uniquely the nurse, standing either literally or figuratively at the bedside, who has the opportunity and the entreé to interact with patients on that spiritual level where they strive to create, love, question, contemplate, and transcend. Here, truly, the nurse is standing on holy ground.

The Nurse as Healer

The nurse, standing as he or she does on the holy ground of caring for the sick, is well situated to be the instrument of God's healing. In the sacred interaction between nurse and patient, the spiritual healing dimension of holistic health care is exemplified and refined. The nurse stands as God's surrogate and as a vehicle for His words and His touch of compassionate care. For the nurse of the Judeo-Christian tradition, spiritually oriented scriptural models of healing abound in both the Old and the New Testaments. Yahweh's healing power is reflected in Old Testament Scripture in such narratives as Elijah's healing of the widow's son (1 Kings 17:17–23) and Elisha's cleansing of Naaman's leprosy (2 Kings 5:1–14). In the New Testament we read that Jesus healed by word and by touch, sometimes even using physical materials such as mud and saliva. Always, Jesus' healings were accompanied by love and compassion for the ill persons or their families, as in the case of Jairus' young daughter, who her parents thought to be dead. Jesus comforted Jairus with the words, "The child is not dead but sleeping" (Mark 5:39). And then, "He took her by the hand and said to her, 'Talitha, cum', which means 'Little Girl, get up!' and immediatly the girl got up and began to walk about" (Mark 5:41). Nurse Theorist Barbara Dossey (1988) identified the characteristics of a nurse healer as having an awareness that "being present" to the patient is as essential as technical skills, respecting and loving all clients regardless of background or personal characteristics, listening actively, being nonjudgmental, and viewing time with clients as times of sharing and serving (p. 42). These characteristics reflect the spiritual nature of healing described in the Old and the New Testament Scriptures.

The Nurse as Wounded Healer

When a nurse is described as a healer, one tends to focus on his or her ability to relieve suffering. The label "healer" evokes the concept of a strong and gifted individual whose ministry is directed by care and compassion; this is an appropriate image. What may be forgotten in such a description is the fact that sometimes the gift of healing has emerged from, and indeed has been honed by, the healer's own experiences of suffering and pain. Henri Nouwen's (1979) classic conceptualization of the wounded healer is most relevant for nurses. Nouwen described the wounded healer as one who must look after personal wounds while at the same time having the ability to heal others. The wounded healer concept is derived from a Talmudic identification of the awaited Messiah:

> He is sitting among the poor covered with wounds. The others unbind all their wounds at the same time and bind them up again, But he unbinds one at a time and binds it up again, saying to himself: "Perhaps I shall be needed; if so, I must always be ready so as not to delay for a moment."
>
> Tractate Sanhedren
> (as cited in Nouwen, 1979, p. 82)

The nurse, as any person who undertakes ministry, brings into the interaction personal and unique wounds. Rather than hindering the therapeutic process, the caregiver's wounds, when not unbound all at once, can become a source of strength, understanding, and empathy when addressing the suffering of others. The nurse as a wounded healer caring for a wounded patient can relate his or her own painful experiences to those of the ill person, thus providing a common ground of experience on which to base the initiation of spiritual care.

A Nursing Theology of Caring: The Nurse's Call

The theology of caring encompasses the concepts of being, listening, and touching and was derived from the author's clinical practice with a variety of acutely and chronically ill patients. The nursing theology of caring is supported by the Christian parable of the Good Samaritan:

> A man was going down from Jerusalem to Jerico and fell
> into the hands of robbers who stripped and beat him and
> went away leaving him half dead . . . a Samaritan came near
> him was moved with pity. He went to him and (bandaged)
> his wounds, having poured oil and wine on them. Then he
> put him on his own animal, brought him to an inn and took
> care of him.
>
> (Luke 10:30, 33–34)

For the nurse practicing spiritual caring as the "Good Samaritan", three key activities may serve as vehicles for the carrying out of the theological mandate to serve the sick: being with patients in their experiences of pain, suffering, or other problems or needs; listening to patients verbally express anxieties or emotions, such as fear, anger, loneliness, depression, or sorrow, which may be hindering the achievement of wellness; and touching patients either physically, emotionally, or spiritually to assure them of their connectedness with others in the family of God.

In and of themselves the acts of being with, listening to, or touching a patient may not constitute spiritual care. These behaviors, however, grounded in a nurse's spiritual philosophy of life such as that articulated in the parable of the Good Samaritan, take on the element of ministry; they constitute the nurse's theology of caring.

Being

An experience with a young cancer patient reflects the importance of being with a patient in need.

A young man, Michael, who was facing mutilating surgery in hope of slowing the progress of advanced rhabdomyosarcoma, asked to talk to me; he said, "I need you to help me understand why this is happening. I need you to help me deal with it." As soon as I sat down, he said, "There are some things I've been thinking about that I need to tell you," and the conversation continued with Michael sharing much about his own faith and his attempt to understand God's will in his life. As I prepared to leave, Michael got up, hugged me, and said, "Our talk has helped a lot"; we prayed together for the coming surgery. Simply being with Michael as he struggled with the diagnosis of cancer in light of his own spirituality constituted the caring. I did not have, nor did I need, any right words; I only needed to be a caring presence in Michael's life.

Emeth and Greenhut (1991), in their discussion of understanding illness, described the importance of being with patients and families, especially when, as with Michael, they need to ask questions for which there are no answers. "We cannot answer the question, 'Where is God in this experience?' for anyone else; rather, we must be willing to be with others in their experience as they live with the questions and wait for their personal answers to emerge. This 'being with' is at the heart of health care" (p. 65).

Listening

The concept of listening is an integral part of being with a person, as was learned from interaction with Michael. However, as his illness progressed, there were also times when being with Michael in silence was a significant dimension of caring. In some situations, however, active listening, with responsive and sensitive feedback to the person speaking, is important in providing spiritual care. Ministering to Philip, a young man diagnosed with anaplastic astrocytoma, revealed the importance of such listening. Philip, because of his neurological condition, had difficulty explaining his thoughts, especially in regard to spiritual matters, yet he very much wanted to talk. Philip described himself as a Born-again Christian, a fact of which he was very proud.

> Philip showed me a well-worn Bible in which he had written comments on favorite Scripture passages. I opened the Bible and focused on a particular passage. Philip's speech was helped by looking at the words. I tried to listen carefully, to follow and comprehend Philip's thoughts on the Scripture and its meaning in his life. Our sharing was validated one day when Philip reached out and took my hand and said, "I'm glad you're here; I really like our talking about God together."

Touching

The Christian Gospel message teaches us compellingly that touch was important to Jesus; it was frequently used in healing and caring interactions with His followers. Loving, empathetic, compassionate touch is perhaps the most vital dimension of a nursing theology of caring. At times the touch may be physical: the laying on of hands, taking of one's hand, holding, gently stroking a forehead; or a nurse's touch may be verbal: a kind and caring greeting, a word of comfort and support.

A rewarding experience with the use of caring touch occurred during an interaction with Erin, a 9-year-old newly diagnosed with acute lymphocytic leukemia.

> Erin was about to begin chemotherapy and was terrified at the thought of having IVs started; the staff asked if I would try to help calm her during the initiation of treatment. One of the pediatric oncology nurses pulled up a stool for me next to Erin so that I could hold and comfort her during the needle insertion. After the procedure was finished and I was preparing to leave, Erin trudged across

the room dragging her IV pole, wrapped her arms around me, and said, "Thank you for helping me to get through that!"

Ultimately the activities of being, listening, and touching, as exemplified in Jesus' parable of the Good Samaritan and in a nursing theology of caring, will be employed in a variety of ways as needed in the clinical setting. This is what constitutes the creativity of nursing practice; this is what constitutes the art of the profession of nursing.

The Nurse's Call: A Nurse's Prayer for Faithfulness

The call is so pure; so uncomplicated;
"Come follow me."
O Lord, I want to follow You; it's all I want, really!
Your voice fills my ears:
sometimes, it's as gentle as a soft breeze
whispering throught the leaves;
other times, it's as powerful as the roar of surf in a
gale force storm.

I want to rush after You, panting and out of breath,
and beg: "I heard Your call to serve Lord; to care for
Your ill and Your infirm. Wait up, please; I'm coming!"
That's what my heart aches for, but you know me so
well, Lord. There's that panic that always creeps in.

I feel like Peter skimming the waves;
suddenly I look down and moan: "I can't do this;
I'm not made for walking on water!"
And, my following You seems to come to a dead halt.

But You're right there with me, Lord;
tenderly stretching out Your hand.
You give me the courage to try again,
with childlike, tottering steps, to come to You.

My legs tremble, and my breath comes in ragged gasps.
The battle has weakened me, but You're so close now.
I know I can make it.

Finallly, I throw myself exhausted into Your waiting
arms, like a long distance runner who's just crossed
the finish line. And the reward is glorious.

Dear Lord, I heard Your call, I chose to follow, I
struggled mightily, You waited patiently,

I'm home.

A Nurse's Prayer for Faithfulness

*We know that all things work together for good for those
who love God, who are called according to His purpose.*

ROMANS 8:28

O God, who called me to this holy ministry, keep
me faithful to my vocation. Help me to make of my
nursing, a prayer of commitment and caring. Let me
recognize every sickroom as a tabernacle where You
dwell. Direct my work that it will become a prayer
of reverence and respect for the sacredness of
human life. Bless me, always, with a grateful heart,
that I may be ever mindful of the precious gift of
serving You in the ill and the infirm. Amen.

References

Dossey, B. M. (1988). Nurse as healer: Toward an inward journey. In B. M. Dossey, L. Keegan, C. E. Guzzetta, & L. G. Kolkmeier (Eds.), *Holistic nursing: A handbook for practice* (pp. 39–54). Rockville, MD: Aspen.

Emeth, E. V., & Greenhut, J. H. (1991). *The wholeness handbook: Care of body, mind and spirit for optimal health.* New York: Continuum.

Nouwen, H. J. (1979). *The wounded healer.* Garden City, NY: Image Books.

Wiederkehr, Sr. M. (1991). *Seasons of your heart.* New York: Harper-Collins.

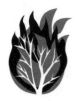

CHAPTER 2

Nursing Assessment of Spiritual Needs

Prove me, O Lord, and try me; test my heart and my mind. For your steadfast love is before my eyes, and I walk in faithfulness to you.

PSALM 26:2-3

Contemplative Nursing

Gentle God,
You alone are the source of my strength
and the center of my life.
how I ache to live those words in my nursing.
But I'm so fragile; so often I forget who You really are.
I keep pretending that I am the source
of my strength and the center of my life, instead of You.
And then, on a bad day, it all starts unraveling.

How can I nurse with gentleness and compassion
in so challenging a health care system?
There are so many complicated issues; they
hinder my caregiving at every turn.
Sometimes I wonder what it is that keeps me going.

But, just when things seem darkest, a tiny
glimmer of light appears.
Gnarled, arthritic fingers seek out my hand
and a small, frail voice whispers to my
heart: "Thank you for being my nurse; God bless you!"

And You do!

For, suddenly, in that fragile moment, I
remember that You, my God, are ever with me;
waiting with outstretched arms and loving embrace.

I remember that You use my hands to touch
with Your tenderness those who are
suffering and sorrowful.
I remember that You use my eyes to look with
Your reverence on those who are rejected and reviled.
I remember that You use my heart to
love with Your love those who are lonely and afraid.

I lay my head gently on Your shoulder and
I bathe in Your nearness. "Don't be afraid,"
You breathe the words into my soul,

"For I am with you always.
Hold tight to my hand and don't let go.
I won't!"

And, now, I remember, again, Dear Lord, that
You are indeed the source of my strength and the
center of my life.

This is the reward of ministering to the sick in Your
Name.

This is the joy of meeting Your Son in caring for the ill
and the infirm.

This is the blessing of contemplative nursing.
Teach me to live and to treasure the gift.

The first step in planning spiritual care for one who is ill is conducting a needs assessment; this may be done formally in the context of developing a care plan, or informally through interaction with the patient and family. The ill individual's level of spiritual development and religious tradition and practice are important variables to be explored. In this chapter a tool to assess spiritual and religious beliefs and needs is presented. Nursing diagnoses related to alterations in spirituality, derived from patient assessment, are also described.

Nursing Assessment of Spiritual Needs

During the past decade JCAHO (the Joint Commission for Accreditation of Healthcare Organizations) has recognized the importance of spiritual and religious beliefs and traditions for persons who are ill or disabled. This concern is reflected in the JCAHO standards relating to spiritual assessment and spiritual care both for those who are hospitalized (Standard R1.1.3.5) and those living in nursing homes (Standard PE1.1.5.1) (Joint Commission For Accreditation of Healthcare Organizations, 2003). The Joint Commission for Accreditation of Healthcare Organizations' standards "reflect the need to recognize and meet the spiritual needs of patients" (Sanders, 2002, p. 107).

The JCAHO website suggests that assessment of patients' spiritual needs should be carried out not only to determine religious denomination, but also to identify spiritual and religious beliefs and practices, especially as related to coping with illness or disability. Some questions to be included in a spiritual assessment include: "Who or what provides the patient with strength and hope?"; "Does the patient use prayer in (his/her) life?"; "What type of spiritual/religious support does the patient desire?"; "What does dying mean to the patient?"; "Is there a role of church/synagogue in the patient's life?"; and "How does faith help the patient cope with illness?" (JCAHO, April 17, 2003).

Nursing assessment of hospitalized patients' problems and needs has become increasingly more sophisticated. Assessment tools vary depending on the care setting, for example, intensive care versus a general care unit; nevertheless, today's nursing assessment instruments are much more detailed than the medical-model–oriented database forms of the past. In addition to assessing physiological parameters, caregivers also assess psychological and sociological factors that may impact patients' illness conditions. A significant weakness, however, among many contemporary nursing assessment tools is the lack of evaluation of a patient's spiritual needs. Frequently, the spiritual assessment is reflected in a single question asking the religious affiliation of the individual. The assumption is that the patient's spiritual care can then be turned over to a hospital chaplain assigned to minister to persons of that religious tradition.

Although the important role of the hospital chaplain is in no way devalued, the nurse, if he or she is to provide holistic care, should have firsthand knowledge of the spiritual practices and needs of a patient. If no detailed spiritual assessment is carried out, such information, even if revealed during a chaplain's visit, might never be communicated to the nursing staff. A patient may, however, reveal a spiritual problem or concern in some depth to the primary nurse during an assessment at the bedside. In health care facilities with well-functioning departments of spiritual ministry, excellent communication often takes place between pastoral caregivers and nursing staff. This is the ideal. In such situations chaplains attend nursing care conferences and share in holistic health planning for patients. If the nursing staff has performed a spiritual assessment, this information, combined with the chaplain's insight and advice, can serve to round out the spiritual dimension of the holistic health care plan.

In the contemporary era of home health care, assessment of a patient's spiritual beliefs and needs is also critical to developing a holistic home nursing care plan. Frequently the home care patient experiencing or recuperating from illness is isolated from sources of spiritual support such as attendance at worship services and interaction with other members of a church or faith group. In such a case, the home health care nurse may be able to assist the patient in verbalizing his or her spiritual or religious needs; the nurse can then offer creative strategies for meeting those needs. The nurse may also provide a bridge between the patient and family and their church, recommending counseling from an ordained pastoral caregiver if this seems warranted.

Spiritual/Faith Development

Central to assessing a patient's spirituality is a basic knowledge of the spiritual development of the human person. A number of theories attempt to track spiritual development; significant among these is James Fowler's paradigm set forth in his book *Stages of Faith Development* (1981).

Fowler (1981) described faith as deeper and more personal than organized religion, as relating to one's transcendent values and relationship with a higher power, or God. Fowler's seven faith stages and their approximate corresponding age categories are as follows:

Undifferentiated Faith, a "prestage" (infancy) in which the seeds of trust, courage, hope, and love are joined to combat such issues as possible "inconsistency and abandonment in the infant's environment" (p. 121). This faith stage has particular relevance for the maternal–infant nurse concerned with issues of parental–infant bonding.

Intuitive–Projective Faith (3–6 years) is an imitative "fantasy-filled" period in which a young child is strongly influenced by "examples, moods, actions and stories of the visible faith of primarily related adults" (p. 133). Pediatric nurses, especially those working with chronically or terminally ill children, will find guidance for dealing with the child's spiritual and emotional needs from Fowler's conceptualization of this stage.

Mythic–Literal Faith (7–12 years) is described as the time when the child begins to internalize "stories, beliefs and observances that symbolize belonging to his or her own faith community" (p. 149). In working with slightly older pediatric patients, the concept of mythic-literal faith can help the nurse to support the child's participation in rites, rituals, and/or worship services of his or her tradition, which may provide support and comfort in illness.

Synthetic–Conventional Faith (13–20 years) describes the adolescent's experiences outside the family unit: at school, at work, with peers, and from the media and religion. Faith provides a "basis for identity and outlook" (p. 172). Fowler's definition of this faith stage provides an understanding of how the ill adolescent may relate to both internal (family) and external (peer) support and interaction during a crisis situation.

Individuative–Reflective Faith (21–30 years) identifies a period during which the young adult begins to claim a faith identity no longer defined by "the composite of one's roles or meanings to others" (p. 182). This is a time of personal creativity and individualism that has important implications for the nurse, including patient autonomy in planning care for the ill young adult patient.

Conjunctive Faith (31–40 years) is a time of opening to the voices of one's "deeper self:" and the development of one's social conscience (p. 198). Nurses caring for patients in this faith stage must be sensitive to the adult's more mature spirituality, especially in relation to finding meaning in his or her illness.

Universalizing Faith (40 years and above) is described by
Fowler as a culmination of the work of all of the previous
faith stages, a time of relating to the "imperatives of absolute
love and justice" toward all humankind (p. 200). Nurses need
to be aware that patients may vary significantly in terms of
degree of accomplishing the imperatives of this final stage.
Assessing approximately where the mature adult patient is,
related to such faith, will help in understanding both the
patient's response to an illness condition and his or her need
for external support in coping with the crisis.

Although a nurse may not be able to identify every patient's
stage of faith development chronologically, Fowler's theory with
its approximate age-associated categorization does present some
guidelines to assist in broadly estimating a patient's level of spiritual development.

The Spiritual Assessment Scale

The author's original standardized instrument to assess adult,
cognitively aware individuals' spiritual beliefs and practices, entitled the "Spiritual Assessment Scale," measures the construct of
Spiritual Well-Being, and contains 21 items, organized into three
subscales: Personal Faith (PF), seven items; Religious Practice
(RP), seven items; and Spiritual Contentment (SC), seven items.
The Spiritual Assessment Scale, which takes approximately three
to four minutes to complete, can be used by practicing nurses in
the health care setting, as well as being employed as a research
instrument. The tool provides nursing staff and nurse researchers
with a broad overview of a patient's personal faith beliefs, the type
of spiritual support he or she receives from religious practices,
and the type and degree of spiritual contentment/distress the
patient is currently experiencing. The 21-item scale is organized
with Likert-type scale response categories (SA—Strongly Agree,
A—Agree, U—Uncertain, D—Disagree, SD—Strongly Disagree)

following each item to facilitate administration; the appropriate categories may be checked by the patient or read aloud and marked by the nurse if a patient is unable to write.*

The construct measured by the Spiritual Assessment Scale, Spiritual Well-Being, includes the dimensions of both spirituality and religiousness, or "religiosity," operationally defined in terms of three discrete concepts: Personal Faith, Religious Practice, and Spiritual Contentment. The term *spiritual well-being* historically emerged following a 1971 White House Conference on Aging. Sociologist of Religion David Moberg (1979) identified spiritual well-being as relating to the "wellness or health of the totality of the inner resources of people, the ultimate concerns around which all other values are focused, the central philosophy of life that guides conduct, and the meaning-giving center of human life which influences all individual and social behavior" (p. 2).

Personal Faith. Personal faith, as a component concept of the spiritual well-being construct, has been described as "a personal relationship with God on whose strength and sureness one can literally stake one's life" (Fatula, 1993, p. 379). Personal faith is a reflection of an individual's transcendent values and philosophy of life.

Religious Practice. Religious practice is primarily operationalized in terms of religious rituals such as attendance at formal group worship services, private prayer and meditation, reading of spiritual books and articles, and/or the carrying out of such activities as volunteer work or almsgiving.

Spiritual Contentment. Spiritual contentment, the opposite of spiritual distress, is likened to spiritual peace (Johnson, 1992), a concept whose correlates include "living in the now of God's love," "accepting the ultimate strength of God," knowledge that all are "children of God," knowing that "God is in control," and "finding peace in God's love and forgiveness" (pp. 12–13). When an individual reports minimal to no notable spiritual distress, he or she may be considered to be in a state of "spiritual contentment."

---

* The Spiritual Assessment Scales does assume belief in a Supreme Being, or God.

Reliability of the SAS

Reliability of the 21-item Spiritual Assessment Scale was determined through administration to a sample population of 179 chronically ill persons who agreed to respond to the tool items for the purpose of statistical analysis. Crumbach's alpha coefficients support reliability of the scale:

Spiritual Assessment Scale (SAS)—21 items
    Alpha coefficient = 0.92

Personal Faith (PF)—7 items
    Alpha coefficient = 0.89

Religious Practice (RP)—7 items
    Alpha coefficient = 0.89

Spiritual Contentment (SC)—7 items
    Alpha coefficient = 0.76

Spiritual Assessment Scale

Instructions: Please check the response category which best identifies your personal belief about the item (response categories: SA—Strongly Agree; A—Agree; U—Uncertain; D—Disagree; SD—Strongly Disagree).

A. Personal Faith

    1. There is a Supreme Being, or God, who created humankind and who cares for all creatures.

       SA _____ A _____ U _____ D _____ SD _____

    2. I am at peace with God.

       SA _____ A _____ U _____ D _____ SD _____

    3. I feel confident that God is watching over me.

       SA _____ A _____ U _____ D _____ SD _____

    4. I receive strength and comfort from my spiritual beliefs.

       SA _____ A _____ U _____ D _____ SD _____

5. I believe that God is interested in all the activities of my life.

SA _____ A _____ U _____ D _____ SD _____

6. I trust that God will take care of the future.

SA _____ A _____ U _____ D _____ SD _____

7. My spiritual beliefs support a positive image of myself and of others, as members of God's family.

SA _____ A _____ U _____ D _____ SD _____

B. Religious Practice

8. Belonging to a church or faith group is an important part of my life.

SA _____ A _____ U _____ D _____ SD _____

9. I am strengthened by participation in religious worship services.

SA _____ A _____ U _____ D _____ SD _____

10. I find satisfaction in religiously motivated activities other than attending worship services, for example, volunteer work or being kind to others.

SA _____ A _____ U _____ D _____ SD _____

11. I am supported by relationships with friends or family members who share my religious beliefs.

SA _____ A _____ U _____ D _____ SD _____

12. I receive comfort and support from a spiritual companion, for example, a pastoral caregiver or friend.

SA _____ A _____ U _____ D _____ SD _____

13. My relationship with God is strengthened by personal prayer.

SA _____ A _____ U _____ D _____ SD _____

14. I am helped to communicate with God by reading or thinking about religious or spiritual things.

SA _____ A _____ U _____ D _____ SD _____

C. Spiritual Contentment

15. I experience pain associated with my spiritual beliefs.

    SA _____ A _____ U _____ D _____ SD _____

16. I feel "far away" from God.

    SA _____ A _____ U _____ D _____ SD _____

17. I am afraid that God might not take care of my needs.

    SA _____ A _____ U _____ D _____ SD _____

18. I have done some things for which I fear God may not forgive me.

    SA _____ A _____ U _____ D _____ SD _____

19. I get angry at God for allowing "bad things" to happen to me, or to people I care about.

    SA _____ A _____ U _____ D _____ SD _____

20. I feel that I have lost God's love.

    SA _____ A _____ U _____ D _____ SD _____

21. I believe that there is no hope of obtaining God's love.

    SA _____ A _____ U _____ D _____ SD _____

Nursing Diagnoses: Alterations in Spiritual Integrity

Nursing diagnoses are currently used in a number of health care facilities to label those patient conditions whose treatment falls within the purview of the nurse. Seven nursing diagnoses related to "alterations in spiritual integrity," which were identified from the author's research (1982a) on spirituality and life threatening illness, include:

"**Spiritual Pain**, as evidenced by expressions of discomfort or suffering relative to one's relationship with God; verbalization of feelings of having a void or lack of spiritual fulfillment, and/or a lack of peace in terms of one's relationship to one's creator" (O'Brien, 1982a, p. 106). A terminally ill patient, experiencing such "spiritual pain," may verbalize a fear that he or she has not lived "according to God's will"; this concern is exacerbated as the possibility of imminent death approaches.

"**Spiritual Alienation**, as evidenced by expressions of loneliness, or the feeling that God seems very far away and remote from one's everyday life; verbalization that one has to depend upon oneself in times of trial or need; and/or a negative attitude toward receiving any comfort or help from God." (O'Brien, 1982a, p. 106). Often, a chronically ill person expresses frustration in terms of closeness to God during sickness; the comment may be heard: "Where is God when I need Him most?"

"**Spiritual Anxiety**, as evidenced by an expression of fear of God's wrath and punishment; fear that God might not take care of one, either immediately or in the future; and/or worry that God is displeased with one's behavior" (O'Brien, 1982a, p. 106). Some cultural groups entertain a concept, although not held by all members of the culture, that illness may be a "punishment" from God for real or imagined faults or failures.

"**Spiritual Guilt**, as evidenced by expressions suggesting that one has failed to do the things which he or she should have done in life, and/or done things which were not pleasing to God; articulation of concerns about the 'kind' of life one has lived" (O'Brien, 1982a, p. 106). Certain individuals, especially those schooled in more fundamentalist religious traditions, experience "guilt" related to their perceived failure to follow God's will, as they understand it. This "guilt" frequently is exacerbated during times of physical or psychological illness.

"**Spiritual Anger**, as evidenced by expressions of frustration, anguish or outrage at God for having allowed illness or other trials; comments about the 'unfairness' of God; and/or negative remarks about institutionalized religion and its ministers or spiritual caregivers" (O'Brien, 1982a, p. 107). Family members of those who are ill may express anger at God for allowing a loved one to suffer.

"**Spiritual Loss**, as evidenced by expression of feelings of having temporarily lost or terminated the love of God; fear that one's relationship with God has been threatened; and/or a feeling of emptiness with regard to spiritual things" (O'Brien, 1982a, p. 107). A sense of "spiritual loss" may frequently be associated with psychological depression; for an individual who feels useless and powerless, there may also be a resultant feeling of alienation from anything or any person perceived as good, such as God.

"**Spiritual Despair**, as evidenced by expressions suggesting that there is no hope of ever having a relationship with God, or of pleasing Him; and/or a feeling that God no longer can or does care for one" (O'Brien, 1982a, p. 107). Although spiritual despair is generally rare among believers, such a diagnosis may be associated with serious psychiatric disorders. If such thoughts or feeling are expressed by a patient, the nurse needs to be alerted, also, to the potential for suicidal ideation or possible behavior.

Of the seven nursing diagnoses related to alterations in spiritual integrity, the one that occurred most pervasively in patient data was that of spiritual pain (O'Brien, 1982a, p. 104).

Although not all nurses may or must feel comfortable in providing spiritual care, the assessment of a patient's spiritual needs is a professional responsibility. Contemporary holistic health care mandates attention to the problems and concerns of the spirit as well as to those of the body and mind. In carrying out an assessment of the patient's spiritual well-being, a nurse may glean information important to supporting the medical and nursing therapies planned for the ill person. Following a spiritual assessment, appropriate spiritual or religious interventions may be provided either by the nurse or through referral to a designated pastoral caregiver.

The Prayer of a Contemplative Caregiver

I came that they may have life and have it abundantly.

JOHN 10:10

O God of magnificence and mystery, what must You be who gifted life with such beauty and such grace. Teach me to contemplate You, through tender care for the sacredness of all human life. Help me to revere the gifts of my ill brothers and sisters; to see in each person a reflection of Your face. Help me to love those I serve in their strengths and in their weaknesses; in caring for them, may I care for You, my Lord and my God. Let my nursing become an unceasing hymn of praise to Your glory, that I may pray with the psalmist:

"O Lord, our God, how awesome is Your Name through all the earth. What are humans that you are mindful of them; mere mortals that You care for them? Yet You have made them little less than a god; crowned them with glory and honor. You have given them rule over the works of Your hands, put all things under their feet ... O Lord, our God, how awesome is Your Name through all the earth" (Psalm 8). Amen.

References

Fatula, M. A. (1993). Faith. In M. Downey (Ed.), *The new dictionary of Catholic spirituality* (pp. 379–390). Collegeville, MN: The Liturgical Press.

Fowler, J. W. (1981). *Stages of faith development.* New York: HarperCollins.

Johnson, R. P. (1992). *Body, mind, spirit: Tapping the healing power within you.* Liguori, MO: Liguori.

Joint Commission for Accreditation of Healthcare Organizations (2003). Spiritual assessment.www.jcaho.org/accredited+organizations/hospitals/standards/hospital+faqs/assessment. 4/17/2003.

Joint Commission for Accreditation of Healthcare Organizations (2003). *Comprehensive accreditation annual for hospitals: The official handbook.* Oakbrook Terrace, Il.: JCAHO.

Moberg, D. O. (1979). The development of social indicators of spiritual wellbeing and quality of life. In D. O. Moberg (Ed.), *Spiritual well-being: Sociological perspectives* (pp. 1–13). Washington, DC: University of America Press.

O'Brien, M. E. (1982a). The need for spiritual integrity. In H. Yura & M. Walsh (Eds.), *Human needs and the nursing process* (Vol. 2, pp. 82–115). Norwalk, CT: Appleton Century Crofts.

Sanders, C. (2002). Challenges for spiritual care-giving in the millennium. *Contemporary Nurse,* 12: 2, p. 107.

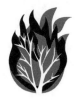

CHAPTER 3

The Nurse-Patient Relationship: A Sacred Covenant

And whoever gives even a cup of cold water . . . [in My Name, will not] lose their reward.

MATTHEW 10:42

The "Cup of Cold Water" Ministry

Only a "cup of cold water," Lord;
it seems like such a small thing?
Yet, to give it in "Your Name," that's
the heart of the message,
Isn't it?

But what does it really mean, Lord,
to give the cup in Your Name?
And to give it to "little ones"; does
that mean to just anyone who
comes along?

I want to minister in "Your Name,"
Lord; that's the desire of my heart.
It's just that some days the fog is so
thick, I can barely see the road.

I need Your help, Dear Lord;

> Please lead me to the place
> where I may give:
> a cup of cold water,
> a bowl of soup,
> a word of comfort,
> a touch of caring,
> in Your Blessed Name.

For centuries the nurse-patient relationship has been unique and individualized. Both patient and nurse bring into the partnership a multiplicity of personal life variables, including such factors as demographics (age, gender, marital status, ethnicity, religion, and socioeconomic status), family history, illness experience, and spiritual orientation. All of the characteristics associated with these variables may impact how the nurse-patient relationship is played out during the course of an interaction.

The Nurse–Patient Covenant

One critical and constant dimension of the nurse-patient relationship relates to the degree of trust engendered between the interacting parties. The element of trust is lived out in most nurse-patient partnerships in terms of a covenant relationship. Although not always formally articulated as such, the presence of an understood covenant between a patient and nurse not only supports the concept of trust between the partners, but also sets up parameters for appropriate *role* behaviors and attitudes. This covenant can be viewed as "sacred" given the nature of the intimacy, indeed the holiness, of the nurse-patient relationship.

The word *covenant* is derived "from the Hebrew word berith, which means 'a binding agreement or pact'" (Senior, 1993, p. 237). The concept of covenant is "one of the Bible's most pervasive means of describing the relationship between God and the community of faith" (Senior, 1993, p. 237). Examples of covenant abound in the Scriptures, beginning with God's covenant with

Abraham in the Old Testament (Genesis 12:1–3). In the Old Testament theology, Yahweh's covenant with Israel "established bonds of loyalty and responsibility between God and humanity" (Boadt, 1984, p. 547). The New Testament covenant relates to Jesus Christ, as the "Son of David and fulfillment of the Messianic prophecies," as depicted in Luke 22:20 (Nowell, 1990, p. 245). A covenant, as envisioned by Henri Nouwen (1991), underlies the spiritual care relationship: "In the covenant there is no condition put on faithfulness. It is the unconditional commitment to be of service" (p. 56).

Many of the covenant-related concepts cited from the theological and pastoral literature have relevance for the nurse-patient relationship:

Bonds of Loyalty and Responsibility—the nurse's commitment to employ all of his or her knowledge and skill to provide the best possible care for the patient; and, in turn, the patient's responsibility to comply, to the best of his or her ability, with the prescribed treatment regimen.

Mutual Obligations—the mutual obligations, on the part of both patient and nurse, to respect and seek to understand the other's attitudes and role behaviors in the context of the nurse–patient relationship.

No Conditions Put on Faithfulness—the nurse will not cease to care lovingly for the patient, regardless of attitudes such as apathy, anger, or even outright noncompliance on the part of a patient.

Not Expecting a Return for Good Services—the degree of the nurse's care and compassion cannot be predicated on the patient's, or family's, gratitude; for physical or emotional reasons, or perhaps both, such thanks may not always be demonstrated.

Isaiah 49:15 provides a moving example of God's covenantal constancy: "Can a mother forget her infant, be without tenderness for the child of her womb, even should she forget, I will never forget you."

Thus, for the nurse called to a ministry of service, whether in nursing practice, nursing education, nursing administration, or nursing research, the theological concept of covenant serves to teach, guide, strengthen, and inspire. The concept of the personal covenantal relationship of God to His people provides a powerful model for the caring and supportive nurse–patient relationships that reflect the art as well as the science of nursing.

The Nurse as "Anonymous Minister"

In addition to the nurse's personal spirituality, a number of other factors are relevant to the spiritual dimension of nurse–patient interactions, including the nurse's comfort level in discussing spiritual issues with patients; the degree of spiritual support provided in the care setting, i.e., support for both patients' and caregivers' spiritual needs; and the emphasis or lack of emphasis on providing spiritual care to patients in the course of professional nursing education. In order to explore, empirically, these questions and issues regarding spirituality and the covenantal nurse–patient relationship, the author conducted focused interviews with 66 contemporary nurses employed in two East Coast metropolitan areas, soliciting individual experiences, attitudes, and behaviors regarding the relationship between spirituality and nursing practice.

A multiplicity of concepts emerged from the interviews associated with such broad areas as nurses' attitudes toward spirituality and spiritual care, the identification of patients' spiritual needs, nursing behaviors regarding the spiritual care of patients, and nurses' perceptions of their roles in ministering to patients' spiritual needs. Ultimately, an overall construct describing the association between spirituality and the nurse-patient relationship emerged from analysis of the interview data and was labeled "The Nurse: The Anonymous Minister."

This construct, which identifies the nurse's frequently unrecognized role in spiritual ministry, consists of three dominant themes: A Sacred Calling, Nonverbalized Theology, and Nursing Liturgy. Each theme incorporates six key concepts reflective of the category's content and orientation (see Table 3.1). This construct, and its supportive themes, reflect a significant conduct of spiritual care among practicing nurses. The study findings explain why at least one author has described nursing as "the finest art" (Donahue, 1985).

TABLE 3.1   The Nurse: The Anonymous Minister

A Sacred Calling	*Nonverbalized Theology*	*Nursing Liturgy*
A Sense of Mission	United in Suffering	Healing Rituals
Messengers of Good Faith	Proddings of the Holy Spirit	Experiencing the Divine
The Almost Sacred	The Day the Lord Has Made	Touching the Core
Touching the Hand of God	Crying for More	Being Present
Sensing the Vibrations	Needing Ventilation	Midwifing the Dying
A Healing Ministry	Praying a Lot	Privileged Moments

The Nurse's Covenant

O God of love and covenant,
I want so much to be like You;
to be gentle,
to be kind,
to be faithful;
to be a small and perfect earthen vessel,
ever available for Your use in my nursing.

But, Dear Lord, I'm so unlike You.
So often I allow myself
to be ungentle,
to be unkind,
to be unfaithful; to be a small and imperfect
earthen vessel, disfigured by cracks on every side.

And my heart breaks, O Lord of my
life, for I fear You could
never choose such an unworthy receptacle
to become a source of
Your love and
Your light for the ill and the infirm.

But, You know that this earthen
vessel is made of clay, Dear
Lord; You who tenderly asked the prophet Jeremiah:
"Can I not do with you as the potter?"

Yes, Lord, God of love and covenant:
You may indeed do with me as the potter.
Remold this scarred and damaged
vessel; remake it into the crucible which
You would have it become.

Let Your light shine forth from this
fragile earthen pot, Dear Lord,
so that the sick who draw from its
contents may know the glorious power of
Your covenant and Your care.

Spiritual Care and Religious Tradition

In order to engage in the assessment of spiritual needs and the
provision of spiritual care for patients whose personal spirituality

is intimately interwoven with religious beliefs and practices, the nurse should have some basic knowledge about the traditions of the major world religions. Obviously, the nurse may not herself subscribe to the religious tenets and practices of a particular patient; however, a broad understanding of the patient's religious culture will assist in identifying spiritual problems and in making referrals to an appropriate pastoral caregiver. The spiritual care of the atheist, who denies the existence of God, and the agnostic, who questions the existence of God, may consist of listening to and providing emotional support for the patient.

This delineation of selected spiritual and religious beliefs and practices may provide the nurse with a starting point in interaction with patients of different faiths. The best strategy, however, in conducting a spiritual assessment is to attempt to learn from the patient or a family member which religious beliefs and practices are most important, especially those pertinent to health and illness issues.

Two major categories of religious tradition are generally considered to be Western spiritual philosophy and Eastern spirituality. The three key Western religions are Judaism, Christianity, and Islam; all are founded on a monotheistic theology. Major Eastern traditions include Buddhism, Hinduism, and Confucianism, the tenets of which differ, especially in regard to the worship of God or of a multiplicity of gods.

Western Religious Traditions

Within the Western religions, Judaism, Christianity, and Islam, the one supreme being is named Yahweh, God, or Allah.

Judaism is described as one of the oldest religions "still practiced in western civilization" and "the foundation on which both Christianity and Islam were built" (Taylor, Lillis, & LeMone, 1997, p. 885). The major religious Jewish groups are Orthodox, Conservative, and Reform; a more recently identified fourth Jewish tradition, which emerged out of a conservative mindset, is

Reconstructionist Judaism (Pawlikowski, 1990, p. 543). The groups differ significantly in regard to religious beliefs and practices. Orthodox Jews follow the traditional religious practices, including careful observance of the Talmudic laws; the Conservative and Reform movements interpret the laws more broadly (Charnes & Moore, 1992). All Jewish traditions emphasize the practice of good deeds or *mitzvahs* each day. Although daily religious rituals are central to the faith of most Jewish persons, health is so valued that "almost all religious injunctions may be lifted to save a life or to relieve suffering" (Charnes & Moore, 1992, p. 66). Jewish people tend to believe that the occurrence of illness is not an accident but rather a time given one to reflect on life and the future (Beck & Goldberg, 1996, p. 16). The keeping of a kosher dietary regimen, if not injurious to health, is very important to many Jewish patients' coping with an illness experience (Fine, 1995), as is the keeping of *Shabbat* or Sabbath, which is observed from sunset on Friday evening to sunset on Saturday. Death, for the Jewish believer, is viewed as part of life; it is important to document the precise hour when death occurs in order to establish the time of mourning, *shiva*, and the annual "honoring of the dead, *Yahrzeit*" (Beck & Goldberg, 1996, p. 18).

Christianity, the largest of the world religions, consists of three main divisions: Roman Catholicism, Eastern Orthodox religions, and the Protestant faiths.

Roman Catholicism identifies that group of Christians who remain in communion with Rome, and who profess allegiance to the doctrines, traditions, philosophies, and practices supported by the pope, as religious leader of the Church. Roman Catholics are trinitarian in theology and place great importance on the seven sacraments: Baptism, Reconciliation (Confession), Holy Eucharist, Confirmation, Matrimony, Holy Orders, and Anointing of the Sick (formerly called "Extreme Unction"); participation in the holy sacrifice of the Mass is the central element of worship.

The Eastern Orthodox tradition, which represents a group of churches whose international leaders are located in Eastern Europe, differs from the Roman Church on both theological issues and aspects of ritual and worship. These churches respect the primacy of the patriarch of Constantinople and include reverence for the Holy Trinity as a central spiritual tenet of the faith. Veneration of holy icons is an important devotion leading ultimately to worship of God the Father, God the Son, and God the Holy Spirit. Currently the term *Eastern Orthodox Church* refers to four ancient patriarchates (Constantinople, Alexandria, Antioch, and Jerusalem), as well as a number of other churches such as those of Russia and Romania, Cyprus, Greece, Egypt, and Syria (Farrugia, 1990, p. 306).

The term *Protestant* generally refers to the churches that originated during the 16th-century Reformation (Gros, 1990). Some characteristics of original Protestantism are "the acceptance of the Bible as the only source of revealed truth, the doctrine of justification by faith alone, and the universal priesthood of all believers" (Livingstone, 1990). Protestant Christians generally regard Baptism and Holy Communion as important sacraments, although denominations may differ on associated rituals. Some of the major Protestant denominations are Adventist, Baptist, Church of the Brethren, Church of the Nazarene, Episcopal (Anglican), Friends (Quakers), Lutheran, Mennonite, Methodist, and Presbyterian.

Christianity is based on the worship of God and promotion of the Kingdom of God through the living out of the Gospel message of Jesus of Nazareth. For the Christian patient, the nurse will need to be sensitive to a multiplicity of religious beliefs and rituals associated with such health-related events as birth, childbearing, organ donation, and death.

Other Western churches of which the practicing nurse should be aware include Christian Science, Church of Jesus Christ of Latter Day Saints (Mormons), Jehovah's Witnesses, and Unitarian Universalist Association of Churches (Taylor, Lillis, & LeMone, 1997, p. 886).

Islam is frequently viewed as having been founded by the prophet Muhammed in the seventh century, with the revelation of the Holy Qur'an. Muslims themselves, however, do not regard Islam as a new religion; "they believe that Allah is the same God who revealed His will to Abraham, Moses, Jesus and Muhammed" (Esposito, 1990). A key tenet of Islam is Tauhid, which means faith in the total Lordship of Allah as ruler of heaven and earth; allied with this concept is the understanding that one's life must be centered on this belief (Abdil-Haqq Muhammad, 1995). Important religious practices for Muslims include the ritual prayer, prayed five times each day (preceded by ritual washing) while facing Mecca (the east); honoring Ramadan, the month of fasting from sunup to sundown, which occurs in the ninth lunar month of the Islamic calendar; and the experience of a hajj, a pilgrimage to Mecca, once in one's lifetime, if possible. Spiritual care for a hospitalized Muslim patient should be focused on providing the time (about 15 minutes) and the setting (a quiet, private place) for the five-times-daily ritual prayer (Kemp, 1996, p. 88). Most hospitals have access to the services of a Muslim spiritual leader, an imam, if requested by the patient.

Eastern Religious Traditions

The major Eastern traditions, Buddhism, Hinduism, and Confucianism, incorporate beliefs about God that differ significantly from those of religions of the Western tradition.

Buddhism derives its beliefs and practices from the life and teachings of the Buddha, the "enlightened one," who lived in India some 2,500 years ago (Borelli, 1990). Myriad Buddhist traditions are associated with the cultures of particular geographical communities, such as Tibetan Buddhism or Chinese Buddhism. Wherever Buddhists are found there are usually monasteries of monks, and sometimes nuns, who preserve the Buddhist teachings and liturgies. Buddhists believe that suffering can be ended by following the eightfold path: "right understanding, right intention, right speech, right action, right livelihood, right effort, right mindfulness and right contemplation" (Borelli, 1990, p. 146). Buddhists do not revere any particular sacraments.

Hinduism does not embrace one particular body of beliefs and practices; the name *Hindu* is derived from the geographical region of the Indus river valley and the subcontinent, Hindustan, where many of those who practice Hinduism reside (Cenkner, 1990). Key concepts in Hinduism relate to reincarnation or rebirth and the idea of *karma*, or "the law by which one's personal deeds determine one's present and future status in this life and in future lives" (Cenkner, 1990, p. 467). Hindus who have lived well do not fear death; it is seen as the preparation for reincarnation into another life.

Confucianism is an Eastern tradition derived primarily from the personal philosophy of the ancient Chinese scholar Confucius. Inherent in Confucian thought is belief in the importance of maintaining harmony and balance in the body. Two potentially conflicting forces are thought to occur in the world, the "yin" and the "yang"; it is critical that these dimensions of function be kept in balance in order to achieve and maintain a good and productive life.

A Model of Spiritual Well-Being in Illness

The midrange nursing theory of spiritual well-being in illness was derived from earlier conceptualizatons in the area of spiritual well-being and also from the nursing model conceived by Joyce Travelbee, in which a central focus of the framework is the concept of finding meaning in an illness experience.

The core component of the nursing theory of spiritual well-being in illness is the concept of finding *spiritual* meaning in the experience of illness. While Travelbee (1971) indeed introduced the importance of spiritual concerns: "the spiritual values a person holds will determine to a great extent his [sic] perception of illness" (p. 16), she never explicitly described the concept of "spiritual well-being" in her model. Rather, Travelbee developed an interactional framework based upon "human-to-human," nurse–patient relationships.

The middle-range theory of sprritual well-being in illness was also inductively derived and concretized through several nursing studies exploring the importance of spiritual well-being in coping with chronic illness and disability. Overwhelmingly positive associations, both quantitatively and qualitatively, were found between spiritual well-being and quality of life. That is, those persons who reported a higher degree of personal faith, spiritual contentment, and religious practice were much more positive about and satisfied with other aspects of their lives and had greater hope for the future, despite sometimes painful and debilitating illnesses.

The key concept of the middle-range theory of spiritual well-being in illness is, of course, that of spiritual well-being itself. In the conceptual model (Figure 3.1), an ill individual is presented as having the ability to find spiritual meaning in the experience of illness, which can ultimately lead to an outcome of spiritual well-being for the sick person. The capacity to find spiritual meaning in an occasion of illness or suffering is influenced by a number of factors. First and foremost, an individual's perception of the spiritual meaning of an illness experience is influenced by personal spiritual and religious attitudes and behaviors. These attitudes and behaviors include variables related to *personal faith*: belief in God, peace in spiritual and religious beliefs, confidence in God's power, strength received from personal faith beliefs, and trust in God's providence; *spiritual contentment*: satisfaction with faith, feeling of closeness to God, lack of fear, reconciliation, security in God's love, and faithfulness; and *religious practice*: support of a faith community, affirmation in worship, encouragement of spiritual companions, consolation from prayer, and communication with God through religious practices.

The impact of these spiritual and religious attitudes and behaviors on one's finding spiritual meaning in illness may also be mediated by such potentially intervening variables as *severity of illness*: degree of functional impairment; *social support*: support of family, friends, and/or caregivers; and current *stressful life events*: emotional, sociocultural, and/or financial.

Figure 3.1 Parish Nursing Practice: A Conceptual Model of Spiritual Well-Being in Illness

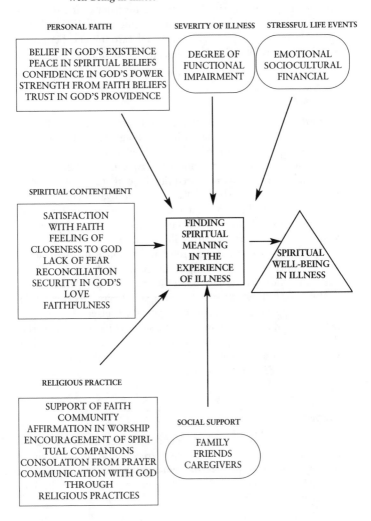

Spiritual and Religious Resources

In order to provide spiritual care to patients from a variety of religious traditions, the nurse must have some familiarity with the available resources, particularly pastoral care, prayer, Scripture, religious rituals, devotional articles, and sacred music.

Pastoral Care

Pastoral care describes the interventions carried out by religious ministers in response to the spiritual or religious needs of others. The activities of the pastoral caregiver, "including sacramental and social ministries, can be as informal as conversational encounters and as formal as highly structured ritual events" (Studzinski, 1993, p. 722). Howard Clinebell (1991), identified five specific pastoral care functions: "healing, sustaining, guiding, reconciling, and nurturing" (p. 43). Such spiritual care interventions may promote significant healing on the part of ill persons.

In making a pastoral care referral, the nurse may contact a priest, minister, rabbi, imam, or other spiritual advisor of the patient's acquaintance and tradition, or refer the patient to a health care facility's department of pastoral care. To facilitate a pastoral care visit, the nurse may prepare a place close to the patient for the spiritual minister to sit, provide privacy to the degree possible in the setting, and cover the bedside table with a white cover if a sacrament such as Anointing of the Sick is to be administered (Taylor, Lillis, & LeMone, 1997, p. 896).

Prayer

The word *prayer* is generally understood as a request or a petition to obtain some good outcome. There are a number of other kinds of prayer, such as prayers of thanksgiving, as well as specific methods of prayer, including vocal prayer, contemplation, and centering prayer.

Although prayer may be engaged in individually by a patient, and often is, it is important to remember that illness, especially acute illness, may create a "barrier to personal prayer" (Shelly & Fish, 1995, pp. 9–10). In such instances a nurse's prayer for and with the patient can be an important spiritual care intervention. Shelly and Fish remind the nurse that his or her prayer should reflect what the patient would pray for if capable of doing so; they advised: "The most helpful prayer is usually a short, simple statement to God of the patient's hopes, fears and needs, and a recognition of God's ability to meet the patient in his [or her] situation" (p. 11). Prayer as a nursing intervention was described by a practicing nurse as "possible in any setting, as long as we ask people's permission" (Mason, 1995, p. 7). Mason believes that prayer can be an important source of peace and comfort for an ill person (p. 7).

Scripture

Scripture, or the "word of God," is written material that represents venerated and guiding principles for many religious traditions. For the Jewish community, the Hebrew Scripture as contained in the Torah represents God's word and laws for his people. For a Christian, both Old (or "First") and New Testaments contained in the Bible are revered. The Old Testament, shared with the Jewish religion, contains "the story of God's work in the world from creation to the period of the second temple (built in 515 BCE)"; the second, or "New Testament . . . begins with the story of Jesus, and contains documents and letters and visions of the early Christian community in the 1st century CE" (Nowell, 1993, p. 857). Other scriptural materials, comforting for patients of the appropriate denominations, might include the Holy Qur'an (for Muslims) or the Book of Mormon (for members of the Church of Jesus Christ of Latter Day Saints).

Shelly and Fish (1988) cautioned that a "principle of appropriate timing" should govern the nurse's use of Scripture (p. 121). If a patient is angry or depressed, or experiencing severe discomfort, such as that accompanying acute pain, the seemingly glib quoting, even of an apparently comforting Scripture passage, may seem like "rubbing salt into the wounds" of the sufferer. If, however, it seems that a patient might benefit from a Scripture passage, the nurse can always ask permission in a noncontrolling manner, leaving the patient free to refuse without discomfort.

When a nurse feels comfortable sharing a passage of Scripture with a patient or family member, the reading can represent an important and valid dimension of spiritual care. Following are some suggested Scripture passages and their underlying messages:

For comfort in times of fear and anxiety—Psalm 23; Philippians 4:4–7; 1 Peter 5:7; Romans 8:38–39.

For fear of approaching death—Psalm 23; John 14:17.

For one in need of healing—Isaiah 53:4–6.

For one seeking God's care and protection—Isaiah 43:2; Isaiah 40:28–31; Psalm 25; Psalm 121; Psalm 139:11–19; Deuteronomy 8:2–3; Jeremiah 29:11; Matthew 10:26–33; Luke 12:22–31.

For one seeking God's mercy and forgiveness—Isaiah 1:18; Isaiah 53:5–6; Hebrews 4:14–16; 1 John 1:9.

For one who is fatigued by illness or life stress—Isaiah 40:31.

Religious Rituals

Religious rituals are sets of behaviors that reflect and honor spiritual or religious beliefs on the part of the participant. There can be a profoundly healing value in participation in religious ritual, especially for the acutely ill person (Texter & Mariscotti, 1994). Thus, the use of or support for religious rituals meaningful to a patient should be an integral part of spiritual care intervention provided by a nurse.

A number of religious rituals may be appropriate for an ill person, whether at home or in the hospital setting. For the Muslim patient whose theology is anchored in the five pillars of Islam, formal prayer (*salat*) is prayed five times daily, facing the east (Mecca). To support the Muslim's daily prayer requirement, a nurse may provide a prayer rug facing the east, situated in a place of privacy, as well as facilities for the ritual washing of hands and face. Advice from an imam may have to be sought regarding fasting if a Muslim falls ill during the holy period of Ramadan. Some other important Muslim rituals are those associated with birth and death. At the birth of an infant the husband stands near his wife's head; when the infant is born the new father whispers a prayer from the Qur'an in the child's ear. Usually a dying Muslim chooses to lie facing Mecca (the east); he or she may also wish to confess prior sins and to recite the words, "There is no God but Allah, and Muhammed is His prophet."

The Orthodox Jewish patient is required to pray three times each day. A male patient, if able, may wish to wear a yarmulke (skull cap) and prayer shawl, as well as phylacteries (symbols of the Ten Commandments) when praying (Charnes & Moore, 1992, p. 66). On the eighth day after birth, a Jewish male child must be circumcised. Circumcision may be done in the hospital, if necessary, or in the home by a *mohel* or Jewish rabbi trained in the procedure. When a Jewish patient is dying, family and friends consider it a religious duty to visit and pray with the dying person and his or her family. In the case of an Orthodox Jew, the nursing personnel may not need to perform postmortem care, as a group from the patient's synagogue, the "burial society," will come to care for the body.

For the Christian person who is ill, the sacraments, as mentioned earlier, as well as prayers particular to each denomination, may be an important part of the healing process. Some years ago, a Roman Catholic could only receive Anointing, then called Extreme Unction, when death was perceived to be imminent. Current Church teaching allows the Catholic patient to request the anointing in the revised ritual of the Sacrament of the Sick at any point during an illness experience. Receiving Holy Communion at that time, or at any time during one's illness, is an important religious ritual for the Catholic and also for many Protestant patients.

Infant Baptism is also an important Roman Catholic ritual. Ordinarily it is carried out in the parish church several weeks after mother and baby have left the hospital. If, however, an infant is in danger of death, any nurse may perform an emergency Baptism by pouring a small amount of water on the child's head and reciting simultaneously, "I baptize you in the name of the Father and of the Son and of the Holy Spirit." Many other Christians practice infant Baptism; some of these church groups include the Episcopal, Lutheran, Methodist, and Presbyterian denominations. Baptismal rites may vary slightly. For example, in the Methodist tradition, "the one baptizing should put his or her hands in the water and then place the wet hand on the baby's head and repeat the baptismal words. In the Lutheran rite, the water is poured on the head three times, while saying the baptismal words" (Reeb & McFarland, 1995, p. 27).

Devotional Articles

Frequently the first clue to an ill patient's religious beliefs and practices is the presence or use of religious or devotional articles. A Jewish person, especially one of the Orthodox tradition, may use a prayer shawl and phylacteries during times of prayer. A Muslim may choose to read passages from the Holy Qur'an, or to pray with prayer beads, which identify the 99 names of Allah. A Christian patient, as well as reading sacred books such as the Bible or the Book of Mormon, will often display devotional items such as relics, medals, crosses, statues, and holy pictures with symbolic meaning for the person. For example, an ill Mexican American of the Christian tradition will frequently carry a medal or picture of Santo Niño de Atocha, a religious personage believed to be instrumental in healing the sick. Other religious symbols an ill person might display include sacred threads tied around the neck of a Hindu, Native American medicine bags, or mustard seeds used by Mediterranean groups to ward off the "evil eye" (Morris & Primomo, 1995, p. 111).

Sacred Music

Music, especially music reflecting an interest in the transcendent, expresses the depth of feeling of one's spirit. Music is a part of all religious traditions, especially as a central dimension of religious worship. Music is frequently used by individuals to relieve stress, and music therapy may be used as an adjunct to healing (Keegan, 1994, p. 169).

Religious music ranges from religious rock, folk, or country-western music, which may appeal to younger patients, to the traditional religious hymns and classical religious pieces such as Handel's Messiah, often preferred by the older generation. Playing a recording of religious music, or even softly singing a hymn with a patient, may be incorporated into spiritual care, if nurse and patient find it meaningful.

This chapter describes the importance of the nurse's role in spiritual care. Many contemporary nurses find assessment, and in some cases intervention, relative to patients' spiritual needs to be a treasured part of their clinical practice. It is nevertheless important to reiterate that not all nurses will feel competent or comfortable undertaking nursing therapeutics in the area of spiritual care. These nurses should, however, be sensitive to the importance of nursing assessment of patients' spiritual needs; referral to a pastoral caregiver for support or intervention is always an acceptable option.

A Nurse's Prayer of Covenant and Caring

I have made a Covenant with my chosen one.

PSALM 89:3

O God of covenant and caring, teach me to reverence relationships. Let me honor the gifts you give so abundantly in the sacred relationships of Your Blessed Trinity. May I revere the blessings of Divine Fatherhood in the person of You, Yahweh, my God; may I treasure the joy of Divine Brotherhood in the person of Jesus; and may I rejoice in the support of Divine Friendship in the person of the Holy Spirit. Help me to model my nursing relationships to reflect Your image and likeness. May I bring to my interactions with those I serve: the parental care of You, God my Father; the passionate love of Your Son, my Lord Jesus; and the inspired wisdom of Your Holy Spirit of understanding and truth. Amen.

References

Abdil-Haqq Muhammad, K. (1995, June). What Muslims believe and why. *Muslim Community News*, 1–2.

Beck, S. E., & Goldberg, E. K. (1996). Jewish beliefs, values and practices: Implications for culturally sensitive nursing care. *Advanced Practice Nursing Quarterly*, 2(2), 15–22.

Boadt, L. (1984). *Reading the old testament: An introduction*. New York: Paulist Press.

Borelli, J. (1990). Buddhism. In J. A. Komonchak, M. Collins, & D. A. Lane (Eds.), *The new dictionary of theology* (pp. 144–147). Collegeville, MN: The Liturgical Press.

Cenkner, W. (1990). Hinduism. In J. A. Komonchak, M. Collins, & D. A. Lane (Eds.), *The new dictionary of theology* (pp. 466–469). Collegeville, MN: The Liturgical Press.

Charnes, L., & Moore, P. (1992). Meeting patients' spiritual needs: The Jewish perspective. *Holistic Nurse Practitioner, 6*(3), 64–72.

Clinebell, H. (1991). *Basic types of pastoral care and counseling.* Nashville, TN: Abington Press.

Donahue, M. P. (1985). *Nursing: The finest art, an illustrated history.* St. Louis, MO: C. V. Mosby.

Esposito, J. L. (1990). Islam. In J. A. Komonchak, M. Collins, & D. A. Lane (Eds.), *The new dictionary of theology* (pp. 527–529). Collegeville, MN: The Liturgical Press.

Farrugia, E. G. (1990). Oriental orthodoxy. In J. A. Komonchak, M. Collins, & D. A. Lane (Eds.), *The new dictionary of theology* (pp. 306–310). Collegeville, MN: The Liturgical Press.

Fine, J. (1995). Long-term care in the Jewish tradition. *The Nursing Spectrum, 5*(22), 2.

Fish, S., & Shelly, J. A. (1988). *Spiritual care: The nurses role.* Downer's Grove, IL: InterVarsity Press.

Gros, J. (1990). Protestantism. In J. A. Komonchak, M. Collins, & D. A. Lane (Eds.), *The new dictionary of theology* (pp. 811–815). Collegeville, MN: The Liturgical Press.

Keegan, L. (1994). *The nurse as healer.* Albany, NY: Delmar.

Kemp, C. (1996). Islamic cultures: Health-care beliefs and practices. *American Journal of Health Behavior, 20*(3), 83–89.

Livingstone, E. A. (1990). *The concise Oxford dictionary of the Christian church.* New York: Oxford University Press.

Mason, C. H. (1995). Prayer as a nursing intervention. *Journal of Christian Nursing, 12*(1), 4–8.

Morris, D. L., & Primomo, J. (1995). Nursing practice with young and middle-aged adults. In W. J. Phipps, V. L. Cassmeyer, J. K. Sands, & Lehman, M. K. (Eds.), *Medical–surgical nursing: Concepts and clinical practice* (5th ed., pp. 45–64). St. Louis, MO: C. V. Mosby.

Nouwen, H. J. M. (1991). *Creative ministry.* New York: Image Books.

Nowell, I. (1990). Covenant. In J. Komonchak, M. Collins, & D. Lane (Eds.), *The new dictionary of theology* (NDT) (pp. 234–246). Collegeville, MN: The Liturgical Press.

Nowell, I. (1993). Scripture. In M. Downey (Ed.), *The new dictionary of Catholic spirituality* (pp. 854–863). Collegeville, MN: The Liturgical Press.

Pawlikowski, J. (1990). Judaism. In J. Komonchak, M. Collins, & D. A. Lane (Eds.), *The new dictionary of theology* (pp. 543–548). Collegeville, MN: The Liturgical Press.

Reeb, R. H., & McFarland, S. T. (1995). Emergency baptism. *Journal of Christian Nursing*, 12(2), 26–27.

Senior, D. (1993). Covenant. In M. Downey (Ed.), *The new dictionary of Catholic spirituality* (NDCS) (pp. 237–238). Collegeville, MN: The Liturgical Press.

Shelly, J. A., & Fish, S. (1988). *Spiritual care: The nurse's role* (3rd ed.). Downer's Grove, IL: InterVarsity Press.

Shelly, J. A., & Fish, S. (1995). Praying with patients. *Journal of Christian Nursing*, 12(1), 9–13.

Studzinski, R. (1993). Pastoral care and counseling. In M. Downey (Ed.), *The new dictionary of Catholic spirituality* (pp. 722–723). Collegeville, MN: The Liturgical Press.

Taylor, C., Lillis, C., & LeMone, P. (1997). *Fundamentals of nursing: The art and science of nursing care* (3rd ed.). Philadelphia: J. B. Lippincott.

Texter, L. A., & Mariscotti, J. M. (1994). From chaos to new life: Ritual enactment in the passage from illness to health. *Journal of Religion and Health*, 33(4), 325–332.

Travelbee, J. (1971). *Interpersonal aspects of nursing* (2nd ed.). Philadelphia: F. A. Davis.

CHAPTER 4

Spiritual Care of the Acutely Ill Person

The Lord will keep you from all evil; he will keep your life.
The Lord will keep your going out and coming in, from
this time on and forevermore.

PSALM 121:7-8

Veronica: A Nurse's Meditation

Standing at the fringes of the crowd,
she feels the restlessness.
She shades her eyes from the hot Jerusalem sun
and peers down the road;
It's so dry and dusty, she can't see anything
but she senses His coming.
Her heart begins to beat fast and her temples pound.
How could they do this to her dear and gentle Rabbi;
the One who taught her to love in His Father's name?

Then, over the rise of a hill, she catches
the first painful glimpse.
The soldiers surround Him; as if He had
the desire, or even the strength to run!
The Cross is fearful; its wood so heavy, its beams so rough.
He can barely drag it down the path; only
the young, strong arms of Simon make
the humiliating procession possible.

As He draws near she sees the beautiful
face; now caked with the dirt of the
streets and blood from the cruel beating.
Crimson droplets trickle into His loving
eyes; her King is crowned with brambles
and thorns, not with gold and jewels.
Her heart breaks and her soul weeps bitter
tears; she feels so helpless.

She has no towel or cloth to wipe the precious
wounded face; only a poor woman's veil,
simple muslin, but soft and clean; put
on that very afternoon to preserve
humility before the eyes of her Lord.
Modesty is no longer relevant; now she must
bare her head to blot the blood and tears
from those same beloved eyes.
She is rewarded with the Blessed image of
the Divine Son of God.

I see him stumble into the ER, leaning
heavily on his comrade's arm.
"He's homeless," his friend from the family
of the streets reports:
"They beat him up, those young punks,
just because he's old."

His body is caked with the dirt of the
streets, and blood from the cruel beating.
His eyes are moist with unshed tears; alive
with the pain of loneliness and fear.
I wash the gentle, weathered face with a
clean, soft towel, and I think of Veronica.
I am rewarded with the Blessed image of the human Son
of God.

The spiritual needs of the adult patient suffering from an acute illness vary greatly depending on such factors as age, religious tradition, and the seriousness of the condition. Acute illness is described by Taylor, Lillis, and LeMone (1997) as "a rapidly occurring illness that runs its course, allowing the person to return to his or her previous level of functioning" (p. 1451).

However, a number of "chronic" disease conditions may also begin or end with an acute illness phase or manifest acute symptoms during periods of exacerbation over the course of the illness trajectory.

During periods of acute illness, whether self-limiting or associated with a chronic disease, the patient may experience significant physical discomfort and anxiety, especially if symptoms are severe or life threatening. Patients with self-limiting illness may need comfort and support in coping with the sequelae of an infectious process, such as the acute pain accompanying a bout with herpes zoster ("shingles"). Individuals experiencing acute exacerbations of a potentially life-threatening chronic illness may need help in coping with the prognosis as well as the diagnosis of their condition.

Spiritual Needs in Acute Illness

Spiritual beliefs and, for some, religious practices, may become more important during illness than at any other time in a person's life. While an individual is enjoying good mental and physical health, spiritual or religious practices may be relegated, in terms of both time and energy, to a small portion of one's life activities. With the onset of acute illness, however, especially if associated with the exacerbation of a chronic condition, some significant life changes may occur both physically and emotionally. First, the ill person is usually forced to dramatically curtail physical activities, especially those associated with formal work or professional involvement. This may leave the individual with a great deal of uncommitted time to ponder the meaning of life and the illness experience. Such a time of forced physical "retreat" may effect considerable emotional change in one's assessment of past and future attitudes and behaviors.

The onset of a sudden and unanticipated acute illness may pose serious emotional and spiritual problems related to fear of possible death or disability. Psychological depression may occur as a result of severe physical symptoms such as acute pain and fatigue. Some patients question God's will and even express anger toward God for allowing the illness to occur. At this point, especially, the nurse must be alert and astute in assessing the spiritual concerns and needs of an acutely ill patient. Although a diagnosis of spiritual distress may be masked by the physical and emotional symptoms of an illness, the patient's remarks can provide a hint as to the presence of spiritual symptoms in need of attention. For example, comments such as "God help me," or "I wonder where God is in all of this?" can give the nurse an opening for informal spiritual assessment.

In essence, meeting the spiritual needs of the acutely ill may encompass basic concepts of spiritual care such as listening, being present, praying or reading Scripture (if acceptable to the patient and comfortable for the nurse), and/or making a referral to a chaplain or other pastoral caregiver. These activities, however, must be handled sensitively, related to the severity of patient symptoms such as pain, nausea, or fatigue. Appropriate spiritual care behaviors for the acutely ill person might include sitting quietly at the patient's bedside for a brief period, saying a short prayer aloud or offering a silent prayer, or sharing a comforting Scripture passage that may help to focus the patient away from the present suffering.

As well as being associated with the acute illness conditions and the acute phases of chronic illness, serious physiological and psychological challenges requiring spiritual support are also present in such experiences as the perioperative journey, the critical care experience, the emergency room experience, and the experience of pain; these are explored in the following sections.

Spiritual Needs of the Perioperative Patient

The term *perioperative* refers to the period encompassing the pre-operative, intraoperative, and postoperative experiences for a surgical patient. Specifically, the preoperative phase begins with the plan to carry out surgery and ends with the actual transfer of the patient to the operating room (OR); the intraoperative phase covers the period of the actual surgical procedure; and the postoperative phase begins with the transfer of the patient out of the OR to recovery, and continues through the healing process to the time of discharge from the physician's care. The perioperative client may be found in a hospital, a community-based surgery center, or, for minor procedures, a physician's office.

The perioperative patient and family may pose significant challenges to the nursing staff related to the anxiety experienced prior to, during, and immediately after the surgery; yet, the perioperative nurse often has little time to develop a relationship with the patient due to the fast-paced nature of the nursing (Dearing, 1997). Some of the most frequently identified causes for fear in the preoperative period are "fear of the unknown," "fear of pain or death," and "fear of changes in body image and self concept" (Taylor, Lillis, & LeMone, 1997, pp. 676–677); fear of the unknown may encompass the other fears. Fear of the unknown may also include fear of the postoperative diagnosis, especially if the surgical procedure is focused on an exploration to determine the possible presence of a malignancy. Fear of surgical death or of a painful postoperative death lurks in the minds of most patients and families during the intraoperative period. Even if the surgery has been described as a "simple procedure," preoperative patients often express fear of "going under the knife" or going under anesthesia, especially if general anesthesia is used.

A dimension of the perioperative nurse's role is to provide comfort and support to patients and families, especially during the pre- and postoperative periods. In a 1994 statement the Association of Operating Room Nurses asserted that "the perioperative nurse designs, coordinates, and delivers care to meet the identified physiologic, psychologic, sociocultural and spiritual needs of patients whose protective reflexes or self-care abilities are potentially compromised because they are having invasive procedures. The nursing activities address the needs and responses of patients and their families or significant others" (cited in Atkinson & Fortunato, 1996, p. 22).

The perioperative nurse can identify a patient's spiritual beliefs through use of the nursing history and thus can provide spiritual care through "acceptance, participation in prayer, or referral to clergy or chaplain" (Taylor, Lillis, & LeMone, 1997, p. 678).

Spiritual Needs of the ICU Patient

In the contemporary critical care unit, with its ever more complex therapeutic technology, the persona of the patient may seem lost in the myriad tubes, wires, and sophisticated monitoring devices. Obviously, a central responsibility of the critical care nurse is to skillfully employ the technology at hand in the service of intensive patient care. If the nurse is to provide truly holistic care to the critically ill patient, however, attention to the needs of the mind and the spirit must accompany the delivery of high-quality physical care. Dossey, Guzzetta, and Kenner, in the introduction to their text *Critical Care Nursing: Body, Mind, Spirit* (1992), admitted that their subtitle may seem inappropriate to some readers who might regard the emphasis on mind and spirit as irrelevant to contemporary science. The authors argued, however, that sensitivity to the patient's emotional and spiritual needs is an essential dimension of the subfield of critical care nursing. They suggested that during a period of critical illness "patients frequently search for how to create new perceptions for their life as well as to find wholeness and spirituality" and that they "need guidance in their transformation" (p. 11). Dossey et al. explained that the critical care nurse, therefore, needs to be sensitive to a variety of factors in order to help patients deal with spiritual issues, including the pluralism of spiritual beliefs and religious practices that patients may adhere to, the difference between spiritual and religious concepts, and the nurse's own possible personal confusion in regard to spiritual or religious values (p. 12).

Virtually all cognitively aware adult patients report significant stress associated with the ICU experience. As well as those discussed already, other identified stressors include "social isolation, enforced immobility, pain from procedures, poor communication with staff, excessive noise and lack of sleep" (Dracup, 1995, pp. 12–13).

Related to the stress of critical illness, with its painful sequelae, as well as the sometimes persistent fear of death and the added stressor of hospitalization in a critical care unit, Busch (1994) recognized that the experience may either enhance or challenge a patient's spiritual or religious beliefs (p. 16). A first step in providing spiritual care for the critically ill patient, then, is to carry out an assessment of the person's spiritual and/or religious beliefs, practices, and current needs. Some pertinent information about spiritual or religious history may be obtained from the patient's chart and from the family; hopefully, information about current spiritual needs will emerge through personal interaction between patient and nurse.

Because of the patient's possible isolation from usual religious practices, such as attending worship services or reading Scripture or other spiritual books, and because of the fear and anxiety about his or her illness condition, the nurse may diagnose spiritual distress in the ICU patient. Twibell, Wieseke, Marine, and Schoger (1996) identified some defining characteristics of a spiritual distress diagnosis for a critically ill patient, including a request of spiritual guidance or support, the verbalization of distress over not being able to carry out usual religious practices, expression of "spiritual emptiness," questioning the credibility of one's belief system, and expressing anger or frustration over the meaning of the present illness experience (p. 249). Following such a diagnosis, the nurse may intervene or may elect to contact a chaplain or other pastoral care provider. Bell (1993) advised that if the nurse chooses to pray with the critically ill patient, using "the patient's own words" in relation to illness-related needs may be comforting (p. 27).

Spiritual Needs of the Emergency Department Patient

An emergency is defined as "any sudden illness or injury that is perceived to be a crisis threatening the physical or psychological well being of a person or a group" (Lazure & DeMartinis, 1997, p. 2501). Although most large hospitals house emergency departments to care for those persons and groups, it is well known that a number of individuals seek care at an emergency room for non-life-threatening, and even routine, problems. This occurs most frequently in large urban inner-city areas, where indigent and homeless individuals have no other available and accessible source of medical care. Nevertheless, the goal of emergency departments is to provide care for the acutely ill and injured.

Spiritual care and support may be an important need for both patient and family in an emergency situation, especially if the admitting diagnosis contains a life-threatening dimension. In 1993, Eileen Corcoran (1993), president of the Emergency Nurses Association, posed the question, "Is it reasonable to believe that the emergency room nurse's role includes addressing spiritual needs of patients and their families?" (p. 183). In posing her rhetorical question in the *Journal of Emergency Nursing*, Corcoran admitted that a significant amount of the ER nurse's time must be spent on meeting the patient's physical needs, but she argued that this does not relieve the ER nurse from attention to spiritual needs. Some suggestions Corcoran offered for spiritual care intervention by emergency nurses include establishing a trusting relationship with the patient; maintaining a supportive environment, including providing privacy for patient and family if necessary and identifying religious resources such as the availability of on-call clergy; and finally, recognizing the role of the nurse in "healing the whole person" (p. 184).

Spiritual Needs of the Patient in Pain

Although no common definition of pain exists, many nurse clinicians still rely on the pragmatic description first articulated in 1968 by McCaffery: "Pain is whatever the experiencing person says it is, existing whenever the experiencing person says it does" (p. 95). A more contemporary, yet also practical, definition identifies pain as "the state in which an individual experiences and reports the presence of severe discomfort or an uncomfortable sensation" (Gunta, 1993, p. 1538). *Pain* is broadly understood as a word used to reflect a subjective perception of distress.

Religious beliefs can be particularly important to the pain experience as they may provide support and strength through such activities as prayer and scripture reading. Religious or spiritual beliefs may also provide the person in pain with a vehicle for finding meaning in suffering, or for "offering" the pain experience to God, in expiation for one's failings or the failings of others. Some individuals, however, may also view pain or suffering as a punishment from God, for example, the concept of *castigo* (punishment) in the Mexican American culture. A nurse or pastor familiar with contemporary theology may be helpful in counseling a patient with this negative perception of God and of the pain experience.

As well as recommending or participating in prayer (if acceptable to the patient in pain) and seeking counsel of a chaplain, another therapeutic spiritual care activity that the nurse may recommend and teach is the use of spiritual imagery (Ferszt & Taylor, 1988). A suggestion that the patient imagine God as a loving parent holding him or her in His arms and gently loving and caring may do much to comfort the person in pain. Some other spiritual care strategies for alleviating patients' pain include listening with a caring manner to the individual's fears and anxieties related to the pain experience, and facilitating the participation of family members or other significant persons who may be a primary source of support.

Spiritual care is an important dimension of holistic care for the person with an acute illness or an acute exacerbation of a chronic condition. Spiritual care is also essential for persons experiencing a serious physical or psychosocial challenge related to a perioperative experience, a critical care experience, an emergency room experience, or a pain experience. Often the nurse must employ creative strategies to intervene spiritually for persons who may be experiencing a crisis of faith as well as a serious illness. Ultimately, however, spiritual care is appropriate and acceptable for the nurse working with acutely ill patients.

A Nurse's Prayer for Devotion

> *I remember the devotion of your youth; / your love as a bride / how you followed me in the desert / in a land unsown.*

>   JEREMIAH 2:2–3

Oh God, who gifted our profession of nursing with the charism of devotion to caring for the sick, teach me to pray. Bless me with the gift of devout and fervent trust, as you lead my patients into the desert of illness or infirmity. Send your Spirit of wisdom and understanding to guide my mind and my heart as I seek to support the fragile bodies and spirits of those who must walk in a "land unsown." Grace my nursing with an enlivened devotion to You, my Lord and my God, that I may share this precious treasure with all whom you have entrusted to my loving care. Amen.

References

Atkinson, L. J., & Fortunato, N. M. (1996). *Berry & Kohn's operating room technique*. St. Louis, MO: Mosby–Yearbook.

Bell, N. (1993). Caring: The essence of critical care nursing. In N. M. Holloway (Ed.), *Nursing the critically ill adult* (4th ed., pp. 14–29). New York: Addison-Wesley.

Busch, K. D. (1994). Psychosocial concepts and the patient's experience with critical illness. In C. M. Hudak, B. M. Gallo, & J. J. Benz (Eds.), *Critical care nursing: A holistic approach* (pp. 8–22). Philadelphia: J. B. Lippincott.

Corcoran, E. (1993). Spirituality: An important aspect of emergency nursing. *Journal of Emergency Nursing, 19*(3), 183–184.

Dearing, L. (1997). Caring for the perioperative client. In P. A. Potter & A. G. Perry (Eds.), *Fundamentals of nursing: Concepts, process and practice* (pp. 1379–1427). St. Louis, MO: C. V. Mosby.

Dossey, B. M., Guzzetta, C. E., & Kenner, C. (1992). Body, mind, spirit. In B. M. Dossey, C. E. Guzzetta, & C. V. Kenner (Eds.), *Critical care nursing: Body, mind, spirit* (pp. 10–16). Philadelphia: B. Lippincott.

Dracup, K. (1995). Key aspects of caring for the acutely ill. In S. G. Funk, E. M. Tornquist, M. T. Champagne, & R. A. Wise (Eds.), *Key aspects of caring for the acutely ill* (pp. 8–22). New York: Springer.

Ferszt, G. G., & Taylor, P. B. (1988). When your patient needs spiritual comfort. *Nursing '88, 18*(4), 48–49.

Gunta, K. E. (1993). Chronic pain. In J. M. Thompson, G. K. McFarland, J. E. Hirsch, & S. N. Tucker (Eds.), *Mosby's clinical nursing* (3rd ed., pp. 1538–1543). St. Louis, MO: C. V. Mosby.

Lazure, L. A., & DeMartinis, J. E. (1997). Basic concepts of emergency care. In J. H. Black & E. Mahassarin-Jacobs (Eds.), *Medical–surgical nursing: Clinical management for continuity of care* (5th ed., pp. 2501–2516). Philadelphia: W. B. Saunders.

McCaffery, M. (1968). *Nursing practice theories related to cognition, bodily pain, and man–environment interaction*. Los Angeles: University of California at Los Angeles.

Taylor, C., Lillis, C., & LeMone, P. (1997). *Fundamentals of nursing: The art and science of nursing care* (3rd ed.). Philadelphia: J. B. Lippincott.

Twibell, R., Wieseke, A., Marine, M., & Schoger, J. (1996). Spiritual and coping needs of critically ill patients: Validation of nursing diagnosis. *Dimensions of Critical Care Nursing*, 15(5), 245–253.

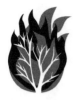

CHAPTER 5

Spiritual Care of the Chronically Ill Person

Those who wait for the Lord shall renew their strength,
they shall mount up with wings like eagles, they shall run
and not be weary, they shall walk and not faint.

ISAIAH 40:31

With Eagle's Wings

Lord God,
The prophet Isaiah taught us the value of hope;
if we but hope in You (Isaiah 40:31),
we will soar as with eagle's wings. (Isaiah 40:31)

That seems such an easy lesson;
only to hope . . . and all will be well.

But when the days are dark,
Dear Lord; when we are
filled with sorrow and suffering,
Isaiah's message seems a
distant echo; a muted bell tolling from afar.
Teach us, Lord God, to hope:
to hope in illness and infirmity;
to hope in pain and anger;

to hope in hurt and frustration;
to hope in anguish and despair.

Guide us to hope in You, O Lord,
that we may indeed, one day,
"soar as with eagle's wings"
in the radiance of Your light and Your love.

For the chronically ill individual, personal spirituality and/or religious beliefs and practices often constitute an important, even critical, dimension of coping with the life changes necessitated by the illness experience. For many persons living with chronic illness, transcendent belief and experience provide the impetus to live and to love in the midst of significant pain and suffering.

Any experience of illness may bring about a degree of disruption in a person's life. Usual patterns of life activity are temporarily, or in some cases permanently, changed or modified to cope with the situation. The need for a major life change occurs more frequently in patients facing chronic illness. Corbin (1996) defined chronic illness as "a medical condition or health problem with associated symptoms or disabilities that require long-term management" (p. 318).

Chronic illness symptoms may range from mild to severe, and often fluctuate between periods of exacerbation and remission. In cases of chronic illness, frequently the fulfillment of previous roles and responsibilities becomes impossible, and significant reorganization of an individual's patterns of behavior is required. Major changes may occur in social relationships and future life plans.

The chronically ill person, although most frequently living at home, may also be found in a hospital or clinic setting; the latter in times of illness exacerbation or during the carrying out of diagnostic or therapeutic procedures. The kind of spiritual care provided by the nurse will be influenced by the setting and also by the type and degree of the patient's disability. Physical disability, such as being unable to ambulate freely, may necessitate a creative strategy to facilitate participation in religious rituals, if desired by the client. Spiritual care may also be directed toward the emotional sequelae of chronic illness, which may affect overall spiritual well-being, such as "low self-esteem, feelings of isolation, powerlessness, hopelessness, and anger" (Soeken & Carson, 1987, p. 606). Spiritual interventions that a nurse can initiate in response are an affirmation of God's love and care for each person, encouragement to participate in rituals shared with others, and support for an individual's hope in God's protection (pp. 608–609).

Spiritual care interventions for the chronically ill are similar to those proposed for the acutely ill patient. They include listening to and being with the patient, which may facilitate the integration of spirituality into coping behaviors; praying with a patient, if the patient so desires; reading Scripture, if appropriate; providing spiritual books or other devotional materials; and referring the patient to a clergy member. These spiritual interventions need to be adapted, however, to particular illness conditions and their sequelae, such as mental illness and physical disability, and to specific settings, such as those involving home health care and homelessness, which are discussed later in this chapter. Obviously, careful attention to the patient's religious tradition should precede any spiritual interventions as well as the assessment of spiritual needs.

Spiritual Needs in Chronic Illness

All individuals have spiritual needs, regardless of religious belief or personal philosophy of life. The experience of illness, especially of a long-term chronic illness, may be a time when spiritual needs previously unnoticed or neglected become apparent (Baldacchino and Draper, 2001). Spiritual needs may manifest in a multiplicity of symptoms, depending on the person's particular theology, religious tradition, or philosophical understanding of the meaning and purpose of life. For the adherent of one of the monotheistic Western religious groups, Judaism, Christianity, or Islam, spiritual needs are generally associated with one's relationship to God.

Some important spiritual needs of chronically ill persons include hope, trust, courage, faith and peace.

Hope

And now, O Lord, what do I wait for? My hope is in you.

PSALM 39:7

Hope, as a general term, relates to an anticipation that something desired will occur. Hope, or the act of hoping, defined theologically for a member of a monotheistic religious tradition, is the "focusing of attention, affectivity and commitment to action toward the future goal of fulfillment in God, the realization of the reign of God" (Hellwig, 1993, p. 506). Shelly and Fish (1988) pointed out that placing one's hope in God does not mean an immediate end to suffering or anxiety; rather, hoping relates to trust in God's support during a crisis (p. 44).

Phillip, a young adult cancer patient who described himself as a born-again Christian, manifested a beautifully direct sense of hope as he faced his illness:

> I put all my hope in Jesus, in the Cross. I have my daily minute with Him. I mean, it's about an hour, but I call it my "minute." I try to always have the special "minutes." I pray to Jesus; He is with me. Jesus is my hope.

Trust

> *I trust in you, O Lord; I say, "You are my God."*
>
> PSALM 31:14

The concept of trust indicates having confidence in something or someone. Theologically, the term is considered to be a relational one, "describing the quality of a relationship among two or more persons" (Schreiter, 1993, p. 982).

In discussing adaptation to chronic illness, nursing scholar Ruth Stoll (1989) noted that "a dynamic spiritual belief system enables us to trust that somehow tomorrow will not be beyond our capacities" (p. 195). Trusting, for the ill person who is a believer, will give a sense of security that God's healing power will be operative in his or her life (Johnson, 1992, p. 92). It is important to recognize, however, that the "healing" that occurs may be of a spiritual or emotional nature, rather than a physical healing.

A recently married and newly diagnosed Burkitt's lymphoma patient, David, spoke eloquently to the concept of trust:

> Well, this is not what I had expected at this time in my life but this is the Cross, the folly of the Cross they say, so I put it in the hands of the "man upstairs." I mean I'm really with Him and He's with me, you know. . . . I have to tell you, though, even with my faith, we're all human, and I was really scared in the beginning. When they first brought me in to the hospital, they rolled me into that ICU, through the doors, and I saw all that equipment and those monitors, I thought: "Whoa! Is this the Cross?" But you know that God is going to be walking beside you.

Courage

> *I took courage, for the hand of the Lord, my God, was upon me.*

> EZRA 7:28

Courage, or emotional strength, is described not as the absence of fear, but rather as "the ability to transcend one's fears, to choose to actively face what needs to be" (Stoll, 1989, p. 196).

Martha, an adult woman in midlife diagnosed with chronic renal failure and experiencing maintenance hemodialysis, spoke openly about the need for courage to face a life dependent on technology:

> You have to get yourself together and face the thing; be courageous about it because nobody is going to do it for you. I think adjusting to kidney failure and dialysis is very difficult because I can't answer why. Why did this happen to me? But my faith says that all things have a reason, and God won't put anything on us that we can't bear. . . . But it's still difficult because chronic illnesses may be with you a long time before they lead to dying; you have to have some courage about it.

Faith

> *Daughter, your faith has healed you.*

> LUKE 8:48

Faith means belief or trust in someone or something. From a theological perspective, faith is the basis of our personal relationship with God "on whose strength and absolute sureness we can literally stake our lives" (Fatula, 1993, p. 379).

An example of the support provided by personal faith in coping with an advanced cancer diagnosis was reflected in Matthew's perception of his condition:

> I can't question how I got this disease or what God's plan is for me. But I know my faith will get me through. At a time like this, faith is the key. My faith makes me strong. Chemo is tough but God's in that too. I don't know; I just know my faith will get me to the place I need to be.

Peace

> *May the Lord give strength to His people, may the Lord bless His people with peace.*
>
> PSALM 29:11

Peace is a sense of being undisturbed, a feeling of freedom from anxiety and fear. Theologically, peace is described as being derived from "a right relationship with God, which entails forgiveness, reconciliation and union" (Dwyer, 1990, p. 749).

A chronic renal failure patient on maintenance hemodialysis described the peace her religious faith afforded her in relation to the disease and treatment regimen. Elizabeth, a two-year veteran of dialytic therapy, reported that the illness experience had a positive effect on her personal spirituality:

> My faith has really strengthened. I'm still a good old "knee-slapping" Baptist. I still love my pastor and I enjoy going to church on Sunday. I pray a lot, but I don't want to ask too much. I'm at peace. If healing is for me, then it will come to me. I just take the attitude that I don't worry about it. God will provide.

Love

> *How precious is your steadfast love, O God.*
>
> PSALM 36:7

To love means to care for or to treasure someone or something. Love, from a religious perspective, relates to "God's benevolent love"; thus, "by association, God's love encompasses human love for God, human love for neighbor, human love for creation, and self-love" (Dreyer, 1993, p. 613).

A cancer patient described the importance of God's love as manifested by her church:

> Well the one thing that helps you deal with this is that you know that your church is behind you. The pastor, he remembers to call you and the church members come to visit and the deacons bring me my Communion to the house. All those things make me feel good; they make me feel loved.

Spiritual Needs of the Mentally Challenged Person

The Person with Mental Illness

Mental health and *mental illness* are relative terms, existing along a continuum of attitude and behavior; the label *mental illness* covers a vast array of diagnostic categories, ranging from mild conditions, such as situational anxiety and depression, to the frank psychosis of schizophrenic disorders. The concepts are culturally determined also. What may be considered pathological in one society, such as the trancelike states entered into during some religious rituals, is normal according to the perception of that particular community.

To assist the nurse in distinguishing a psychiatric client's spiritual needs from those directly related to his or her mental health condition, John (1983) suggested a series of questions relating to such issues as whether a person's religious belief or behavior seems to contribute to the illness, whether religious concerns reflect a pathological inner conflict, whether religious beliefs and behavior bring comfort or distress, and whether religion is used merely as a context for psychotic delusions (pp. 81–83). In the case of a religiously oriented delusion, the role of the person providing spiritual care is to "support the person but not the delusion" (Wagner, 1992, p. 156).

Specific spiritual care interventions for the psychiatric client will vary greatly, depending not only on the patient's identified needs, but also on personal spiritual and religious history. For this patient population, especially, the nurse will need to employ the art, as well as the science, of nursing.

Attempting to analyze and understand the spiritual needs of a mentally ill patient, especially a depressed individual, is extremely challenging to the nurse. Much time may be spent in simply encouraging the patient to verbalize his or her concerns. During the interaction, however, the nurse can communicate a sense of care and empathy, sometimes opening the door to the possibility of therapeutic intervention in the area of spiritual need.

The Cognitively Impaired Client

Cognitive functioning affects both physical and psychosocial dimensions of an individual's life. Although cognition is "primarily an intellectual and perceptual process, [it is] closely integrated with . . . emotional and spiritual values" (Arnold, 1996, p. 977). The cognitively disabled person may have been diagnosed from infancy with some degree or type of mental retardation; cognitive processes may have been injured during childhood or early to middle adulthood as a result of illness or traumatic injury; or a cognitive disability may have its onset only in the elder years, in cases such as senile dementia.

In the past, the religious community has raised some concern as to the role of the cognitively disabled individual in the church or worship setting. Some have questioned whether a person who is not cognitively functional can have a relationship with God, much less understand the meaning of religious practices. Reverend John Swinton (1997), a minister and former psychiatric–mental health nurse, argued, however, that "faith is not an intellectual exercise but relational reality," and that relationship to God is for any of us a mystery beyond intellectual understanding (pp. 21–22). True affective understanding of God, Swinton concluded, occurs at a much more interior level than that of intellectual comprehension (p. 23). Swinton's position is supported by ethicist Stanley Hauerwas (1995), who pointed out that, although including cognitively handicapped persons in worship services may not be easy, the extent to which they may bring about the unexpected is a reminder that "the God we worship is not easily domesticated" (p. 60). Hauerwas contended that "in worship the church is made vulnerable to a God who would rule this world not by coercion but by the unpredictability of love" (p. 60).

A magnificent example of spiritual care for the profoundly cognitively impaired is that carried out in L'Arche (the Ark) communities founded by French Canadian philosopher Jean Vanier. Vanier (1975) began his work during a visit to the small town of Trosly, France, when he moved into a house with two mentally handicapped men. Gradually, other mentally challenged persons began to come, together with volunteers to live with and care for them. New L'Arche communities started to flourish under Vanier's spiritual philosophy of responsibility to care for one's brothers and sisters; this caring was to be done as in a family, where all are accepted and equal as God's children. Henri Nouwen, who spent his later years living in a L'Arche community in Canada, wrote, "Today, L'Arche is a word that inspires thousands of people all over the world . . . its vision is a source of hope" (1988, p. 13).

Spiritual Needs of the Physically Disabled Client

Who are those persons on whom our society imposes the label "disabled"? Theologian Michael Downey (1993) believes that, excluding those who may temporarily require special attention such as infants and young children, the very elderly, and persons incapacitated for a time due to illness or accident, the term disabled generally describes individuals who are to some degree permanently impaired (p. 273). Downey defined the disabled as those persons "whose capacities of mind or body are diminished in any way during the pre, peri or post natal period or at some later period in the course of psychosomatic development, so as to necessitate particular attention or special assistance in meeting basic human needs" (1993, p. 273).

Disability may affect all dimensions of an individual's life: physical, social, emotional, and spiritual. The goal of rehabilitation is to return to the disabled person as much preillness functioning in each of those life arenas as possible. Ultimately the goal of the rehabilitation process is to help an individual regain as much independence as possible. Theologian Donald Senior (1995) pointed out that although an authentic response would be to bear the illness in a "spirit of Faith," persons with disabilities need spiritual support in the process of achieving fullness of life (p. 17). The concept of spiritual care is thus an appropriate dimension of rehabilitation nursing. Some suggested spiritual interventions for a disabled patient experiencing rehabilitation are recommending a spiritual counselor; providing prayer materials, as denominationally appropriate; and introducing imagery, music, or meditative prayer to the client (Solimine & Hoeman, 1996, p. 636). In regard to the latter activity, Solimine and Hoeman suggested that through prayer, disabled individuals are able to give over their situation to God and "trade their weakness for God's strength" (p. 631). Accardi (1990) suggested three other pastoral care interventions for the disabled: listening to the patient's "spiritually significant stories," that is, walking with the patient on his or her spiritual journey; "indwelling the stories," or expressing the empathy and compassion that results from entering into another's pain; and "linking the stories" with biblical references that may help the person find meaning in, or the ability to transcend, the disability (p. 91).

Spiritual Needs of the Client in the Community

Spiritual care of the client in the community is carried out in the overall context of community health nursing. In discussing the role of the community health nurse in providing spiritual care to clients, Burkhardt and Nagai-Jacobson (1985) advised that three questions may guide the initial assessment of need: Does the client's formal religious tradition or denomination provide a good structure for spiritual care?; Does the way in which the client speaks or does not speak of God reveal spiritual concerns or needs?; and Do the client's religious contacts seem to provide strength and comfort? (p. 194). The answers to such questions can then lead the nurse to a more detailed spiritual assessment and plans for intervention, if needed.

The Home Health Care Client

Spiritual assessment and, if appropriate, the provision of spiritual care, are important activities for the home health nurse, as "hope and faith" have been identified as playing a major role in the home care client's adaptation to illness or disability (Rice, 1996, p. 47). Jaffe and Skidmore-Roth (1993) suggested several issues to be addressed in a spiritual assessment of the home health care patient: religious beliefs and practice, how one's belief (or lack of belief) in a supreme being relates to illness, specific people who provide spiritual support, religious symbols of importance (e.g., a Bible or Sabbath candles), religious restrictions (dietary, medical treatment), requirements for church attendance, and religious leaders (pp. 42–43). Bauer and Barron (1995) noted that spiritual nursing interventions are particularly important for the elderly client who lives alone in the community with no religiously based support system available; the community health nurse may be the only visitor who is able and willing to discuss spiritual issues with such a client.

Spiritual Needs of the Homeless Client

Homelessness has been defined by the federal government as "the absence of 'fixed, regular and adequate nighttime residence' "; this statement also encompasses the use of public or private shelters for sleeping (Virvan, 1996, p. 1025). Earlier in the century, the homeless were conceptualized primarily as derelicts of society; recently, a new homeless population consisting of women and children and families has emerged within urban communities (Vernon, 1997, p. 484). Fontaine (1995a) identified four subgroups of homeless people: the chronically mentally ill, individuals who abuse illegal drugs, teens living on the streets, and families with children (pp. 472–473). These homeless persons often lack not only shelter, but also adequate food, clothing, and health care.

What constitutes spiritual care of the homeless client who is poor? Murray (1993) described the spiritual care of homeless men as moving beyond the basic needs of food and shelter, and involving such activities as providing the men with unconditional acceptance and speaking with them in a caring manner; providing small devotional materials supportive of spiritual practices that can be carried out privately; planning religious services that are supportive rather than condemning; and praying with a person if acceptable (p. 34). In a study of homeless women, Shuler, Gelberg, and Brown (1994) found that the use of prayer among clients was significantly associated with decreased alcohol and drug abuse, fewer worries, and less depression (p. 106). The authors also suggested the use of spiritual reading materials, such as religious books or the Bible, and clergy counseling, which together with the use of prayer can decrease the effects of stressful stimuli and increase coping strategies (p. 112).

Personal spirituality and/or religious beliefs and practices may constitute an important mediating variable for the individual coping with a chronic illness. For the chronically ill patient, such concepts as hope, trust, courage, and love may take on new and deeper meaning following the illness onset. Nurses may support and facilitate the presence of positive attitudes and attributes in a patient's life through a variety of spiritual care interventions. As well as providing spiritual care for the hospitalized patient, contemporary nurses need to be sensitive to the spiritual needs and concerns of persons with a variety of other chronic conditions and in a variety of settings.

A Nurse's Prayer for a Place of Silence

> There's so much noise, Dear Lord,
> and so much pain;
> and so very many wounds needing to be healed.
> Some days it almost overwhelms me.
>
> I yearn to be alone with You
> in a place of silence;
> I long to fill my ears with the
> whisperings of Your Holy Spirit;
> I ache to immerse my heart in
> the compassion of Your care.
>
> In the midst of my hectic nursing
> days, I thirst for an oasis of solitude, where my
> parched soul can be quenched with
> the living waters of Your love.
> I hunger for a banquet of peace
> where my starving spirit can

be nourished with the
tender quiet of Your love.
Free me, O Lord, from the prison
of my frantic activity;
extricate me from the binds of my overcrowded
schedule; liberate me from the constraint
of my anxious thoughts.

Lead me, gently, O Lord, to that
sacred place of silence,
hidden in the recesses of
the human heart.
For, it is there that You dwell,
Dear Lord;
it is there that you enfold
my vulnerability with
Your strength;
it is there that You teach me
the true art of compassionate caring.

Mentor my nursing, O Lord, in the
quietness of Your love.

References

Accardi, R. F. (1990). Rehabilitation: Dreams lost, dreams found. In H. Hayes & C. J. van der Poel (Eds.), *Health care ministry: A handbook for chaplains* (pp. 88–92). New York: Paulist Press.

Arnold, E. N. (1996). The journey clouded by cognitive disorders. In V. B. Carson & E. N. Arnold (Eds.), *Mental health nursing: The nurse–patient journey* (pp. 977–1019). Philadelphia: W. B. Saunders.

Baldacchino, D. and Draper, P. (2001). Spiritual coping strategies: A review of the nursing research literature. *Journal of Advanced Nursing*, 34(6), 833–841.

Bauer, T., & Barron, C.R. (1995) Nursing interventions for spiritual care. *Journal of Holistic Nursing*, 13(3), 268–279.

Burkhardt, M. A., & Nagai-Jacobson, M. G. (1985). Dealing with spiritual concerns of clients in the community. *Journal of Community Health Nursing*, 2(4), 191–198.

Corbin, J. (1996). Chronic illness. In S. C. Smeltzer & B. G. Bare (Eds.), *Brunner and Suddarth's textbook of medical–surgical nursing* (8th ed., pp. 317–324). Philadelphia: J. B. Lippincott.

Downey, M. (1993). Disability: The disabled. In M. Downey (Ed.), *The new dictionary of Catholic spirituality* (pp. 273–274). Collegeville, MN: The Liturgical Press.

Dreyer, E. (1993). Love. In M. Downey (Ed.), *The new dictionary of Catholic spirituality* (pp. 612–622). Collegeville, MN: The Liturgical Press.

Dwyer, J. A. (1990). Peace. In J. A. Komonchak, M. Collins, & D. A. Lane (Eds.), *The new dictionary of theology* (pp. 748–753). Collegeville, MN: The Liturgical Press.

Fatula, M. A. (1993). Faith. In M. Downey (Ed.), *The new dictionary of Catholic spirituality* (pp. 379–390). Collegeville, MN: The Liturgical Press.

Fontaine, K. L. (1995a). Contemporary issues: AIDS and homelessness. In K. L. Fontaine & J. S. Fletcher (Eds.), *Essentials of mental health nursing* (3rd ed., pp. 467–477). New York: Addison-Wesley.

Hauerwas, S. (1995). The church and mentally handicapped persons: A continuing challenge to the imagination. In M. Bishop (Ed.), *Religion as a disability: Essays in scripture, theology and ethics* (pp. 46–64). Kansas City, MO: Sheed & Ward.

Hellwig, M. K. (1993). Hope. In M. Downey (Ed.), *The new dictionary of Catholic spirituality* (pp. 506–515). Collegeville, MN: The Liturgical Press.

Jaffe, M. S., & Skidmore-Roth, L. (1993). *Home health nursing care plans*. St. Louis, MO: C. V. Mosby.

John, S. D. (1983). Assessing spiritual needs. In J. A. Shelly & S. D. John (Eds.), *Spiritual dimensions of mental health* (pp. 73–84). Downers Grove, IL: InterVarsity Press.

Johnson, R. P. (1992). *Body, mind, spirit: Tapping the healing power within you.* Liguori, MO: Liguori Publications.

Murray, R. (1993). Spiritual care of homeless men: What helps and what hinders? *Journal of Christian Nursing, 10*(2), 30–34.

Nouwen, H. (1988). *The road to daybreak: A spiritual journey.* New York: Doubleday.

Rice, R. (1996). Developing the plan of care and documentation. In R. Rice (Ed.), *Home health nursing practice, concepts and application* (pp. 41–60). St. Louis, MO: C. V. Mosby.

Schreiter, R. (1993). Trust. In M. Downey (Ed.), *The new dictionary of Catholic spirituality* (pp. 982–983). Collegeville, MN: The Liturgical Press.

Senior, D. (1995). Beware of the Canaanite woman: Disability and the Bible. In M. Bishop (Ed.), *Religion and disability: Essays in scripture, theology and ethics* (pp. 1–26). Kansas City, MO: Sheed & Ward.

Shelly, J. A., & Fish. S. (1988). *Spiritual care: The nurse's role* (3rd. ed.). Downers Grove, IL: InterVarsity Press.

Shuler, P. A., Gelberg, L., & Brown, M. (1994). The effects of spiritual religious practices on spiritual well-being among inner city homeless women. *Nurse Practitioner Forum, 5*(2), 106–113.

Soeken, K. L., & Carson, V. B. (1987). Responding to the spiritual needs of the chronically ill. *Nursing Clinics of North America, 22*(3), 603–611.

Solimine, M. A., & Hoeman, S. P. (1996). Spirituality: A rehabilitation perspective. In S. P. Hoeman (Ed.), *Rehabilitation nursing: Process and application* (2nd ed., pp. 628–643). St. Louis, MO: C. V. Mosby.

Stoll, R. I. (1989). Spirituality and chronic illness. In V. B. Carson (Ed.), *Spiritual dimensions of nursing practice* (pp. 180–216). Philadelphia: W. B. Saunders.

Swinton, J. (1997). Restoring the image: Spirituality, faith and cognitive disability. *Journal of Religion and Health, 36*(1), 21–27.

Taylor, C., Lillis, C., & LeMone, P. (1997). *Fundamentals of nursing: The art and science of nursing care* (3rd ed). Philadelphia: J. B. Lippincott.

Vanier, J. (1975). *Be not afraid*. New York: Paulist Press.

Vernon, J. A. (1997). Basic human needs: Individual and family. In P. A. Potter & A. G. Perry (Eds.), *Fundamentals of nursing: Concepts, process and practice* (4th ed., pp. 478–495). St. Louis, MO: C. V. Mosby.

Virvan, D. (1996). The journey marked by homelessness. In V. B. Carson & E. N. Arnold (Eds.), *Mental health nursing: The nurse–patient journey* (pp. 1023–1038). Philadelphia: W. B. Saunders.

Wagner, W. (1992). The voices on psychiatry: Inner tumult and the quest for meaning. In L. E. Holst (Ed.), *Hospital ministry: The role of the chaplain today* (pp. 151–162). New York: Crossroad.

CHAPTER 6

Spiritual Care of the Ill Child

He took her by the hand and called out, Child, get up! Her spirit returned she got up at once.

LUKE 8:54-55

All the Towns and the Villages

Dear Lord Jesus,
You are the role model for all nurses.
You didn't minister only in the Synagogue;
You went out to the "cities and the villages"
(Matthew 9:35);
You went to wherever the ill and the
infirm were in need.

You went to Capernaum and cleansed the
man with the unclean spirit (Luke 4:35);
You went to the home of Simon and visited
his feverish mother-in-law (Luke 4:39);
You went to Lake Gennesaret, and touched
a leper (Luke 5:13);
You went to Gallilee and healed a paralytic
(Luke 5:24-25);
You went to meet a Centurian and cured
his servant (Luke 7:10);
and You went to the house of Jairus and
restored his daughter (Luke 8:34).

Dearest Lord Jesus,
You taught:
"Daughter your faith has made you well."
(Luke 8:48);
You counseled:
"Those who are well have no need of a physician,"
but the sick do. (Luke 5:31);
You advocated:
"Her sins… have been forgiven, [because] she has
shown great love" (Luke 7:47);
and, You referred:
"I will ask the Father and he will give you another
Advocate to be with you forever, the Spirit of Truth"
(John 14:16).

Teach me, Dear Lord, to learn from
Your Blessed example.

Perhaps no therapeutic intervention calls on the nurse's creative skills as much as that of providing spiritual care to an ill child. Children are unique and challenging in their varied developmental stages; as frequently noted, a child is much more than a small adult. Children, especially ill children, tend to be astoundingly straightforward in expressing their questions and concerns. They expect no less from their caregivers. Honesty and directness, to the degree possible and appropriate, is the most therapeutic approach for a nurse in the provision of spiritual care to an ill child.

The comments of a pediatric nurse practitioner well describe pediatric spiritual care:

> Working with children you have to have a very clear sense
> of your own spirituality, because they are very sensitive to
> the spiritual in others. You have to have a spirituality that
> projects total acceptance because, if not, the kids can read

right through it; anything that's a facade or put on, they know it in a heartbeat. . . . In my nursing with children and families I have learned a lot about spiritual needs. You just need to be open and give them the chance. They're not afraid of the hard questions, like "what's it like to die?" or "will I die?"; but you have to not be afraid to let them ask. Children will give you spiritual clues; you just have to pick up on them.

The Ill Child and Religious Practices

For a child of any religious tradition who is experiencing illness, the ability to participate in religious devotions or practices, such as prayer, may provide a source of comfort and stability. Religious practices and beliefs can impact a child's health; illness may be interpreted in light of a child's religious understanding (Spector & Spertac, 1990, p. 58). The presence in a sickroom of devotional articles such as holy pictures, statues, crucifixes, crosses, or Bibles may provide a sense of security and stability during the disruption of usual life activities. For the preschooler who has a concrete concept of God as protector and father, simple bedtime prayers such as "Now I lay me down to sleep, I pray the Lord my soul to keep," may help the child to feel more at ease during the night. The reading of a religious story or looking at images from a children's picture Bible can be comforting. If mealtime grace is usual in the family, this may be carried out in the sickroom. A preschooler, ill during a religious holiday such as Christmas, Easter, or Hanukkah, should be encouraged to participate in as many of the associated rituals as possible, to help maintain some sense of normalcy in the child's life.

In the case of an ill school-age child, use of a Bible or prayer book, if part of one's tradition, can be encouraged. A Jewish child may want to experience the lighting of Sabbath candles on Friday evening and have traditional passages from Hebrew Scripture read to him or her. The early school-age child can be encouraged to pray, but will, as noted earlier, expect to have prayers answered, so some counseling may need to be done around that issue. The older school-age child will have learned that prayers are not always directly answered; thus a discussion about the meaning of prayer will be helpful. Some school-age children find it important when ill to continue to participate in certain religious practices such as reception of the sacraments (Holy Eucharist and the Sacrament of Reconciliation), also. Special religious anniversaries, Christmas, Easter, Rosh Hashanah, Yom Kippur, Hanukkah, Ramadan, may be very important to the school-age child, especially if participation in the associated worship rituals is usual in the family. Some reflections of the religious meaning of the celebrations may be brought into the child's sickroom, for example, the setting up of a small Christmas crèche, or a menorah. These spiritual symbols can help the child cope with the frightening nature of an illness experience.

The ill adolescent may need spiritual counseling about the relationship of his or her sickness to the religious or spiritual meaning of life. During this developmental period, when the teen may question many of the tenets of organized religion, the young person might well question "why me?" in relation to an illness. The adolescent who has a strong commitment to his or her church and has experienced consistent participation in activities such as weekly Sunday school, church youth group, youth choir, or Bible study group may experience significant anxiety over not being able to participate in these activities, which are social as well as religious. Visits from an adolescent's peers in such a church group can provide support and comfort, as well as distracting the teen from the illness experience. Adolescence is also a time when young people cherish privacy. Teens often choose to keep their deepest and most treasured feelings to themselves. Thus, adolescents may "reject formal worship services, but engage in individual worship in the privacy of their rooms" (Wong, 1997, p. 472). It is important, even in illness, to allow for such periods of privacy, to the degree possible, for an adolescent patient.

Pediatric head nurse Judith Van Heukelem-Still (1984) wrote that, in assessing the spiritual needs of children, it is important not only to ask questions but also to observe the child for unusual behaviors such as nightmares or withdrawal from social activities (p. 5). She pointed out that the kind of visitors and cards a child receives may give some hint of whether spiritual influences and support are present (p. 5).

Spiritual Needs of the Acutely Ill Child

The child experiencing an acute illness, even if being cared for at home, may suffer psychosocial sequelae such as loneliness related to isolation from a peer group and interruption of school and school-related social activities (Melamed & Bush, 1985). For the older school-age child or adolescent, missing classes may cause not only a sense of alienation from peers, but also anxiety about future goals related to college and career. The adolescent may worry about "keeping up" with classes, even in the case of a relatively temporary condition. The ill teen whose schoolwork has been interrupted may feel some anger at God or at religious beliefs and question "Why me?" Spiritual counseling at such a time will allow the adolescent to verbalize frustration and potentially achieve a degree of peace and patience, a sense that ultimately all will be well.

The Hospitalized Child

The hospitalized child is generally experiencing an acute illness or an acute exacerbation of a chronic condition. Such factors as the severity of illness, type of care unit (e.g., pediatric intensive care unit versus general pediatric care unit), previous hospital experience, and family support will influence the child's emotional and spiritual needs. Ashwill and Volz (1997) identified some universal stressors for the hospitalized child, however, including separation from family, fear of pain or physical injury, and fear of the unknown. The spiritual care of the child should include spiritual support of the parents. In discussing spiritual ministry in a pediatric unit, Arnold (1992) asserted that pediatric ministry must include the entire family (p. 94). Because, Arnold noted, hospitalization of a child represents a crisis situation, needs are usually identified in spiritual language: "hope, trust, love and acceptance"; such needs may be met through the use of religious resources or simply by developing caring relationships with the child and family (p. 95).

Spiritual Needs of the Chronically Ill Child

Childhood chronic illness is a long-term condition for which there is no cure, and which may impact the child's physical and psychological functioning. Statistics suggest that 10–15 percent of the pediatric population is chronically ill (Martin, 1997). Management of a child's chronic illness is complicated because of the necessity of family involvement in the provision of care (Johnson, 1985). A situation of childhood chronic illness may interfere in sibling relationships because parental attention is often heavily focused on the sick child. Although some non-ill siblings cope well, jealousy and emotional distress can occur for the well child (Holiday, 1989); the situation may thus engender feelings of guilt and inadequacy in the chronically ill sibling.

Fulton and Moore (1995) believe that the spiritual well-being of the school-age child with a chronic illness significantly impacts the course of illness and treatment (p. 224). They described two nursing approaches to providing spiritual care as "therapeutic play," to generate understanding of the child's perception of spirituality vis-à-vis the illness experience; "bibliotherapy," employing such techniques as storytelling or journaling to help the child explore the meaning of life; and "use of self" in establishing rapport that may comfort the child and decrease anxiety associated with the illness and treatment (pp. 228–231).

Spiritual Needs of the Dying Child

Like other ill children, the dying child's spiritual needs are reflective of age, spiritual or religious background, and degree of physiological and cognitive functioning. As a rule, the broad needs of dying children model those of dying adults; they desire comfort and freedom from pain, and the security that they will not be alone at the time of death (Martin, 1997, p. 414). These needs, Martin added, will be more acutely manifested in the school-age child and the adolescent (p. 414). Four of the most frequently occurring emotional reactions of dying children are "fear, depression, guilt and anger" (Winkelstein, 1989, p. 231). A school-age child, especially, may experience fear related not so much to the death itself but rather to the dying process. Children of this age may have witnessed the deaths of older family members or friends and are fearful of having to go through the pain and suffering they observed. The preschooler can feel guilty about dying, and leaving parents and siblings; he or she may feel responsible for the illness. The dying adolescent, while also experiencing some degree of fear and guilt, frequently goes through a period of depression and anger over the illness and impending death. As noted earlier, adolescence is the time of questioning spiritual and religious beliefs, as well as being the developmental stage when privacy is valued. Thus the dying adolescent may internalize and hide feelings of anger and depression for some time, resulting in an unexpected eruption of emotion as death nears. The nurse must be sensitive to the age-related developmental stage of the child and also keep in mind that children can "see through" dishonesty and subterfuge quite easily; they find security in truth and directness, even if the information is painful. Caregivers must remember as well that a dying child who has experienced significant contact with the health care system may be very knowledgeable about his or her disease; such children expect information at a level of sophistication that may seem far beyond that warranted by chronological age.

Pediatric oncologist Kate Faulkner (1997) offered some general suggestions related to caring for a dying child; these include being flexible in one's approach, being sensitive to the use of nonverbal communication, respecting the child's desire for privacy, and being "explicit and literal" in responding to questions about death (p. 69). These maxims are most appropriate for the provision of spiritual care. Regardless of a dying child's age and religious tradition, a nurse needs to employ the art as well as the science of nursing in approaching such difficult topics as spirituality and death. Perhaps the best advice is to let the child take the lead, through questions or comments; the nurse can then attempt to cross over, as it were, to the child's world, to that place where the dying child may feel alone. Thus the nurse can become friend and advocate, as well as spiritual caregiver.

A pediatric oncology nurse described the difficulty and the rewards of such nursing advocacy:

> In peds oncology, the most stressful time is around a child's death, and it's the most rewarding time also. It's a gifted experience to be with that child and family. It's a lot like being a midwife to send the child to God; but it hurts so much to lose them when you've become their friend and the family's friend. But it's a spiritual experience for the nurse and for the child. Sometimes you pray with them, sometimes you sing hymns with them, and then again, maybe you just hold them.

Spiritual Needs of the Family of the Ill Child

Certainly not to be neglected in the case of a dying child are the spiritual needs of the family, those of both parents and healthy siblings. As in caring for the child, a nurse will need to call on all of his or her own spiritual strength and experience in order to journey with a family during the predeath and death experience. Cook (1982) suggested, first, that one accept that the family members are probably "not totally rational" during this time (p. 125). Second, Cook advised that the family be encouraged to "continue to function as a family," and that family communication be fostered (p. 125). A parent of a dying child may express seemingly undue anger over a small "glitch" in the provision of hospital or hospice nursing care; this is related to the terrible frustration associated with the loss of parental control in protecting one's child. Nonjudgmental, caring support expressed by a nurse during such an outburst may go far in alleviating the parent's anxiety. The family may also experience internal disorganization during the terminal illness and death of a child. With the ill child receiving so much attention, well siblings can experience feelings of neglect and rejection. Well siblings may also feel guilty about being healthy while a brother or sister is suffering from catastrophic illness. A supportive nurse who welcomes the verbalization of fears and anxieties on the part of all members of the family can facilitate communication between parents and well children.

Children have unique and important spiritual needs in dealing with illness and disability. For the young child as well as for the teen, the support of personal faith and religious practice can significantly mediate the suffering involved with an illness experience. Families of children who are ill also need and benefit from spiritual care.

A Nurse's Prayer for the Gifts of the Spirit

> *The Advocate, the holy Spirit, whom the Father will send
> ... will teach you everything, and remind you of all that [I]
> (Jesus) have said to you.*

JOHN 14:26

Come, Holy Spirit, and grace me with the openness
to hear your voice and to do your will. Bless my
nursing with Your sacred gifts:
grant me wisdom in making clinical assessments;
understanding in listening to patients' needs; knowledge for carrying out therapeutic interventions;
right judgment in identifying illness symptoms;
courage in implementing aggressive therapies; reverence in supporting patient and family concerns; and
wonder and awe at seeing Your presence in each
person for whom I care. Teach me, dear Holy Spirit,
to be to all I serve, a vessel of your love. Amen.

References

Arnold, J. (1992). The voices on pediatrics: Walking with children
    and parents. In L. E. Holst (Ed.), *Hospital ministry: The role of
    the chaplain today* (pp. 93–106). New York: Crossroad.

Ashwill, J. W., & Volz, D. (1997). The ill child in the hospital and
    other care settings. In J.W. Ashwill & S.C. Droske (Eds.),
    Nursing care of children: Principles and practice (pp. 346–371)
    Philadelphia: W.B. Saunders.

Cook, M. (1982). Ministering to dying children and their families. In
    J. A. Shelly (Ed.), *The spiritual needs of children* (pp. 117–129).
    Downers Grove, IL: InterVarsity Press.

Faulkner, K. W. (1997). Talking about death with a dying child.
    American Journal of Nursing, 97(6), 64–69.

Fulton, R. A., & Moore, C. M. (1995). Spiritual care of the school age child with a chronic condition. *Journal of Pediatric Nursing*, 10(4), 224–231.

Holiday, B. (1989). The family with a chronically ill child: An interactional perspective. In C. L. Gilliss, B. M. Highley, B. M. Roberts, & I. M. Martinson (Eds.), *Toward a science of family nursing* (pp. 300–311). New York: Addison-Wesley.

Johnson, S. B. (1985). The family and the child with chronic illness. In D. C. Turk & R. D. Kerns (Eds.), *Health, illness and families: A life-span perspective* (pp. 110–154). New York: John Wiley & Sons.

Martin, G. T. (1997). The child with a chronic or terminal illness. In J. W. Ashwill & S. C. Droske (Eds.), *Nursing care of children: Principles and practice* (pp. 394–417). Philadelphia: W. B. Saunders.

Melamed, B.G., & Bush, J.P. (1985). Family factors in children with acute illness. In D.C. Turk & R.D. Kerns (Eds.), *Health, illness and families: A lifespan perspective* (pp. 183–219). New York: John Wiley & Sons.

Spector, R. E., & Spertac, A. M. (1990). Social and cultural influences on the child. In S. R. Mott, S. R. James, & A. M. Spertac (Eds.), *Nursing care of children and families* (2nd ed., pp. 53–75). New York: Addison-Wesley.

Van Heukelem-Still, J. (1984). How to assess spiritual needs of children and their families. *Journal of Christian Nursing*, 1(1), 4–6.

Winkelstein, M. (1989). Spirituality and the death of a child. In V. B. Carson (Ed.), *Spiritual dimensions of nursing practice* (pp. 217–253). Philadelphia: W. B. Saunders.

Wong, D. L. (1997). *Whaley & Wong's essentials of pediatric nursing* (5th ed.). St. Louis, MO: C. V. Mosby.

CHAPTER 7

Spiritual Care of Families

Bear one another's burdens, and in this way you will fulfill the law of Christ.

GALATIANS 6:2

Bear One Another's Burdens

Dear Lord Jesus,
the apostle Paul taught that
Your followers should "bear one another's
burdens" (Galatians 6:2).
Those who do so, he promised, would fulfill Your law.

But how can I take on "another's burdens" when I
already have so many of my own, Dear Lord?

What if I help another, and no one helps me?
That's the frightening part of
this teaching, Lord Jesus;
Will I have more burdens than I can bear?

But . . . You have taught that
in giving, I will receive;
in grieving for others, I will be comforted;
in being merciful, I will be shown mercy;
and in becoming poor in spirit,

I will inherit the kingdom of heaven
(Matthew 5:3–10).
Grant me the courage, and the
strength, and the love to bear another's burdens
and so fulfill the law of the Lord.

The family is an important resource in the provision of spiritual care, not only for the sick child but for the ill adult as well. There are a number of understandings of the term family in contemporary society. Generally, the concept evokes an image of the basic nuclear family composed of two legally married parents and one or more offspring. Friedmann (1992) defined *family* as "two or more persons who are joined together by bonds of sharing and emotional closeness, who identify themselves as being part of the family" (p. 9). Today, however, there is a growing emergence of the single-parent family; for the single, unmarried individual, a number of persons belonging to such associations as church or friendship groups may be loosely described as family.

The family plays an important role in managing its members' health: primary prevention in supporting a healthy lifestyle, secondary prevention related to decisions to treat illness symptoms, and tertiary prevention manifested by family support of a member's compliance with a prescribed therapeutic regimen (Danielson, Hamel-Bissell, & Winstead-Fry, 1993, p. 11).

The Family, Illness, and Spirituality

Because healthy families generally function as units, it is important to minister to the spiritual needs of the entire family when one member is ill or in need of support (Clinebell, 1991). Families faced with serious short-term or chronic long-term illness of one of the members can benefit greatly from spiritual support provided by friends, church members, or pastoral care providers both within or outside the health care system. Thus, the nurse should welcome a family's presence as a resource in the provision of spiritual support; including family members in a religious ritual or prayer service may help them feel comfortable in sharing in the spiritual support and care of the ill person (Peterson & Potter, 1997, p. 452). Research has identified prayer and belief in God as being the most important coping strategies for a family dealing with illness (Friedmann, 1992, p. 331).

The family's particular spiritual or religious tradition and experience will, of course, direct the kind and degree of spiritual care and support that will prove helpful during an illness experience. For the family not of a religious tradition, spiritual care may consist simply of the presence and concern demonstrated by those providing the intervention. For the family whose members are or have been actively involved in a church or faith group, the religious prayers and practices of the community can be extremely comforting. A Jewish family may appreciate reading the Psalms or other passages found in the Jewish canon of Scripture; for the Muslim family, a passage from the Holy Qur'an can provide support and comfort; and for the Christian family, the Gospel messages of Jesus often provide hope and sustenance during times of illness.

Spiritual Needs of the Family in Acute Illness

Families of acutely ill patients can be found both at home and in the hospital. Because of the unexpected and often sudden onset of an acute illness, or of an acute exacerbation of a chronic condition, families may be neglected and left to fend for themselves regardless of the setting. In a home care situation, where the family is more directly involved in a therapeutic regimen, spiritual support of extended family members and friends can be available and accessible; in the hospital a more formal type of spiritual care may be required. In the hospital setting, however, many families feel constrained by the institution's restrictions and schedules (Katonah, 1991). Most hospital and clinic waiting rooms abound with anxious family members in need of spiritual support. Some needs identified by the families of acutely ill persons include the desire for competent care, pain management, compassion, and extended family support in coping with the impact of the illness on their lives (Durand, 1993, p. xii). Additional needs perceived by the families of hospitalized acutely ill patients are information about changes in a patient's condition and honest answers to questions (Leavitt, 1989, pp. 266–267). Lynn-McHale and Smith (1993) described religion as an "additional support for families experiencing crisis" and considered addressing a family's spiritual and religious concerns as facilitating coping in an acute illness experience (p. 318).

The Family in the Intensive Care Unit

Clark and Heindenreich (1995) identified spiritual well-being for the acutely ill patient experiencing intensive care as encompassing the support of caregivers, family members and friends, and religion and faith beliefs. The family of an acutely ill patient hospitalized in an intensive care unit (ICU) may spend long hours in waiting rooms, sometimes rarely leaving the hospital setting. This is a time when the arrival of a chaplain or nurse willing to provide spiritual care is generally welcomed unequivocally. Families need to verbalize their anxieties to someone with a caring heart as they attempt to face the severity of a loved one's illness. Families of ICU patients often express feelings of helplessness and isolation due to restricted visiting hours in a unit; the nurse or chaplain who is able to spend even a brief period of time with the family can become a bridge between the professional/technical aspects of the intensive care environment and the caring dimensions of the health care facility. Ultimately, spiritual support is reported to be a key dimension of family care in the ICU (Rukholm, Bailey, & Coutu-Wakulczyk, 1991).

Some spiritual care interventions for the family in a critical care setting might include giving information about the patient, environment, and staff, to the degree possible; encouraging the family to verbalize their anxieties and concerns; suggesting some coping strategies for attempting to keep up with physical needs such as nutrition and sleep; and reinforcing the fact that the family's anxiety is normal in such a situation, with the suggestion of some possible coping strategies to reduce stress (Gillman, Gable-Rodriguez, Sutherland, & Whitacre, 1996, p. 15).

Spiritual Needs of the Family in Chronic Illness

Chronic illness may have periods of acute exacerbation, requiring intense medical care and perhaps even hospitalization. Because of the long-term nature of chronic illness, families may become very fatigued and frustrated in the process of providing care. The family of a chronically ill person must continually be alert to changes in the health of their loved one; thus, these families need "ongoing support from friends, health care providers and communities" (Gilliss, Rose, Hallburg, & Martinson, 1989, p. 289).

Often, following a chronic illness diagnosis, both the patient's and the family's lives are disrupted because of a treatment regimen involving surgery and possible chemotherapy. The family needs significant spiritual support to facilitate coping with the myriad illness-related life changes (Sproull, 1992, p. 125).

In a study of 101 cancer patients and 45 parents of children with cancer, Spilka, Spangler, and Nelson (1983) discovered that spiritual and religious support was more important than psychological counseling; some activities appreciated were prayer, religious or spiritual reading, discussing church-related issues, spiritual counseling, and simply the presence of the spiritual caregiver (pp. 101–102). And, Raleigh (1992), in a study comparing 45 cancer patients and 45 patients with other chronic illnesses, found that overall the most important sources of hope were family, friends, and religion.

Spiritual Needs of the Family Coping With a Terminal Illness

The spiritual needs of the family of an adult who has entered into the dying process are discussed in Chapter 9. Here, a brief discussion of family needs in the predeath phase is presented; a case example is drawn from the author's research with family members of terminally ill persons.

In exploring the concept of nurse–family spiritual relationships among 11 hospice nurses and 12 bereaved families, Stiles (1990) identified five behaviors ascribed to nurses: being, doing, knowing, receiving and giving, and welcoming a stranger (p. 235). A nurse's way of being is sitting with and listening to the family; doing includes explaining, reassuring, and comforting; knowing involves sensitivity to the dying process; receiving and giving describes quality time spent between nurse and patient; and welcoming a stranger means inviting the patient's family to help prepare for the death (pp. 237–243). Wright (1997) asserted that listening to and being present to witness a terminally ill patient's and family's suffering is "the soul" of clinical nursing with families (p. 3). A veteran of 20 years of clinical work with families, Wright (1997) maintained that concern about a family's religious and spiritual beliefs has been one of the "most neglected" topics in family care. Yet, she asserted "the experience of suffering becomes transposed to one of spirituality as family members try to make meaning out of their suffering and distress" (p. 5).

Nora, whose 42-year-old son Matthew was terminally ill, asserted:

> It's only God and people's prayers that's getting me through this; they are holding me up. People have been sending prayers in cards and with phone calls. My wonderful priest is praying all the time. I don't know how I could survive without this spiritual support.

Nora admitted that sometimes she became angry with God over Matt's illness and questioned why, but she concluded, "Even when I was screaming at God, because you know, why, and why, and why? Even when I was angry with Him, I knew that God was crying with me" (O'Brien, 1992, p. 67).

Spiritual Needs of the Homeless Family

Only in recent years have texts dealing with family care begun to include the plight of the homeless family. Although families have been the last subcategory to be added to the American cadre of homeless persons, they are now considered to be "the most rapidly growing segment of the [homeless] population" (Friedmann, 1992, p. 109).

Providing spiritual care to homeless families, from a nursing perspective, will require all of the art, creativity, and spiritual strength a nurse can muster during a health care encounter. Because of the transient nature of the homeless, nurses may experience only brief and intermittent interactions with them. Because of the stigma and embarrassment of the homeless condition, parents seeking emergency or clinic care for themselves or their children may be shy about expressing their anxieties and concerns with a nurse caregiver; children, and especially teens, may also be reticent to discuss the pain associated with their homelessness.

An important strategy for the nurse is to provide a welcoming, accepting, and respectful environment for the homeless family seeking care. A compassionate and nonjudgmental attitude can go far in supporting the homeless client's fragile self-concept and may allow the opportunity for some spiritual sharing between client and nurse. If this occurs, the nurse may be able to guide the family in finding religious, and possibly some material, support to assist them in coping with the suffering associated with homelessness.

Although the patient as the center of attention often receives much spiritual support and care, the patient's family members may be neglected or forgotten. Nurses have a prime opportunity to minister spiritually to family members, especially during critical or terminal illness. Perhaps the most elusive category of families for the nurse to reach are those experiencing homelessness. The nurse must employ art and creativity in attempting to provide spiritual intervention for this sometimes neglected population.

A Nurse's Prayer for Courage in Suffering

I have said this to you, so that you may have peace in me. In the world you will face persecution, But take COURAGE; I have conquered the world.

JOHN 16:33

Lord Jesus, wounded healer of our hearts, teach me to embrace suffering. This is not an easy prayer; I get very afraid. Sometimes it seems "my soul is sorrowful unto death" (Matthew 26: 38). Only You whose "sweat became as drops of blood falling on the ground" can be my teacher and my guide. I don't understand sickness and sorrow. I hurt with those in pain; I want to take away their suffering. I long to cry out with You "Father, if You are willing, take this cup away." Bless me, Lord Jesus, with the courage and the love to complete Your prayer: "still not my will but Yours be done" (Luke 22: 39–42). Amen.

References

Clark, C., & Heindenreich, T. (1995). Spiritual care for the critically ill. *American Journal of Critical Care*, 4(1), 77–81.

Clinebell, H. (1991). *Basic types of pastoral care and counseling.* Nashville, TN: Abington Press.

Danielson, C. B., Hamel-Bissell, B., & Winstead-Fry, P. (1993). *Families, health & illness: Perspectives on coping and intervention.* St. Louis, MO: C. V. Mosby.

Durand, B. A. (1993). Preface: Determination of need. In S. L. Feetham, S. B. Meister, J. M. Bell, & C. L. Gillis (Eds.), *The nursing of families* (pp. ix–xiii). Newburg Park, CA: Sage.

Friedmann, M. M. (1992). *Family nursing: Theory and practice.* (3rd ed.) Norwalk, CT: Appleton & Lange.

Gilliss, C. L., Rose, D., Hallburg, J. C., & Martinson, I. M. (1989). The family and chronic illness. In C. L. Gilliss, B. M. Highley, B. M. Roberts, & I. M. Martinson (Eds.), *Toward a science of family nursing* (pp. 287–299). New York: Addison-Wesley.

Gillman, J., Gable-Rodriguez, J., Sutherland, M., & Whitacre, J. H. (1996). Pastoral care in a critical care setting. *Critical Care Nursing Quarterly*, 19(1), 10–20.

Katonah, J. (1991). Hospitalization: A rite of passage. In L.E. Holst (Ed.), *Hospital ministry: The role of the chaplin today* (pp. 55–67). New York: Crossroad.

Leavitt, M. B. (1989). Transition to illness: The family in the hospital. In C. L. Gilliss, B. M. Highley, B. M. Roberts, & I. M. Martinson (Eds.), *Toward a science of family nursing* (pp. 161–186). New York: Addison-Wesley.

Lynn-McHale, D. J., & Smith, A. (1993). Comprehensive assessment of families of the critically ill. In G. D. Wegner & R. J. Alexander (Eds.), *Readings in family nursing* (pp. 309–311). Philadelphia: J. B. Lippincott.

O'Brien, M. E. (1992). *Living with HIV: Experiment in Courage.* Westport, CT: Auburn House.

Peterson, V., & Potter, P. A. (1997). Spiritual health. In P. A. Potter & A. G. Perry (Eds.), *Fundamentals of nursing: Concepts, process and practice* (pp. 440–456). St. Louis, MO: C. V. Mosby.

Raleigh, E. D. (1992). Sources of hope in chronic illness. *Oncology Nursing Forum, 19*(2), 443–448.

Rukholm, E. E., Bailey, P. H., & Coutu-Wakulczyk, G. (1991). Family needs and anxieties in the ICU. *The Canadian Journal of Nursing Research, 23*(3), 67–81.

Spilka, B., Spangler, J. D., & Nelson, C. B. (1983). Spiritual support in life threatening illness. *Journal of Religion and Health, 22*(2), 98–104.

Sproull, A. (1992). The voices on cancer care: A lens unfocused and narrowed. In L. E. Holst (Ed.), *Hospital ministry: The role of the chaplain today*. New York: Crossroad.

Stiles, M. K. (1990). The shining stranger: Nurse–family spiritual relationships. *Cancer Nursing, 13*(4), 235–245.

Wright, L. M. (1997). Spirituality and suffering: The soul of clinical work with families. *Journal of Family Nursing, 3*(1), 3–14.

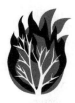

CHAPTER 8

Spiritual Care
of the Older Adult

*Even to your old age I am he, even when you turn gray I
will carry you. I have made, and I will bear; I will carry
and will save.*

ISAIAH 46:4

Compassionate Caregiving

Sitting humbly amidst His followers,
on a Galilean hillside,
He taught of compassionate caregiving;
The Carpenter of Nazareth, the Lamb of God, the
Savior of the world, who promised:
"Whatever you do for my least ones, you do for me!"

His lesson is so simple;
His message so caring:
give some food to those who are hungry;
give a drink to someone who's thirsty;
welcome strangers; dress people who need clothes;
visit your brothers and sisters who can't get out;
and take care of the sick.

"I've not had as much time as
I'd like to pray lately, Dear God,"
a geriatric nurse whispers, as she tenderly lifts a spoonful
of soup to the lips of a frail elder.

"Dear Lord, if only I could fit more scripture reading into my life," an ICU nurse prays, as he solicitously places some ice chips on the parched tongue of a newly extubated patient.

"I'd love to spend more hours in church with You, Dear Lord," an ER nurse implores, as she compassionately helps a homeless stranger onto a waiting gurney.

"Dear Lord, even when I pray I sometimes feel far away from You," a recovery room nurse admits, as he caringly piles warm blankets on a shivering post-op patient.

"I want to visit with You much more in prayer, Dear Lord," a home care nurse muses, as she lovingly comforts a disabled patient in his loneliness.

"Dear God, I wish I knew how to pray better," a hospital staff nurse longs, as he gently wraps a blood-pressure cuff around the trembling arm of a new admission.

The Lord replies to His nurses: "I treasure your desire for intimacy with me; it must always be so, but remember also that I am the hungry elder to whom you tenderly feed a cup of soup; I am the thirsty ICU patient whose parched tongue you solicitously moisten;
I am the homeless stranger you compassionately welcome to your ER; I am the shivering post-op patient you caringly clothe;
I am the homebound person you lovingly visit;
and, It is my trembling arm round which you gently wrap your blood-pressure cuff.
It is I, dear nurse, for whom you care, and in that caring, your nursing is blessed with the gift of My Presence.
In that caring, your nursing becomes your prayer;
and I accept it with joy."

Current definitions of the older patient based on chronological age are changing as a result of the increasing longevity and functional ability of contemporary men and women. In a study to determine the preferred group descriptor of older Americans, the terms *mature*, *older*, and *senior* were the most frequently chosen adjectives; *aged* and *old* were the most disliked terms (Finley, 1989, p. 6). Demographic profiles identify persons as older adults if they have passed the age of 65. Individuals between 65 and 74 years of age are described as "young old"; those over 74 are identified as the "older elderly."

More and more older adults, especially in the younger-old category, are remaining in the workforce or initiating second or third careers; many are also involved in full-time volunteer activities. Ultimately, Finch (1993) posited, the aging process may become a time of peace and joy during which the elder, no longer struggling with the challenges of career or ego, may be able to enjoy the beauties of loved ones and of nature in "wise tranquility" (p. 11). Wisdom is a spiritual gift that the older adult has to give to the world, a gift much needed in contemporary society.

Spirituality and the Older Adult

Scholars of aging disagree as to whether the older adult becomes more or less involved in both spiritual and religious issues (Bianchi, 1995; Burt, 1992). Admittedly, some of the physical and psychosocial deficits of older age may hinder one's religious practice; however, personal spirituality often deepens. If an older person is relatively well, research has shown that religious practice may increase. Membership in a church "is claimed by 73% of women and 63% of men older than 50 years, although fewer attend regularly" (Roen, 1997, p. 356); older adults tend to view the practice of religion as more important than do younger adults (Peterson & Potter, 1997). A church or synagogue may provide social networks for an older adult, as well as delineating a structure within which to live out one's spiritual beliefs. Some church groups may even facilitate health care for the older adult through the support of a parish nurse, as discussed in Chapter 10.

In order to provide spiritual care to an older adult, it is important for the caregiver to have some understanding of the developmental faith tasks of aging. One useful paradigm is that of James Fowler's (1981) stages of faith development (discussed in Chapter 2). To explain the late adult era, the final two of Fowler's stages are appropriate: Conjunctive Faith, stage 5, and movement toward stage 6, Universalizing Faith. Stage 5, or Conjunctive Faith (midlife and beyond), is a time of attempting to look beyond rational explanations and seeing their limitations. In this stage, the older adult may look back on earlier religious beliefs and traditions, which may have been discarded, and begin to reincorporate them into current attitudes and practice. Fowler called this a "reclaiming or reworking of one's past" (1981, p. 197).

Fowler's sixth stage, Universalizing Faith, occurring in the final years of life, is identified as rare: "The persons best described by it have generated faith compositions . . . inclusive of all being" (1981, p. 200). Persons in the sixth faith stage possess "enlarged visions of universal community."

Religious Practice

As an outgrowth of and support for one's spiritual development, religious practices may be very important to the quality of life of an older adult. The religious or faith tradition of the elder will direct the nature of specific practices. Studies of religiosity among elders have, however, identified certain practices common to a number of religious denominations. Some of these include prayer and meditation, church membership, participation in religious worship services, study of religious doctrine, and spiritual reading.

The religious practice universally identified with most Western and Eastern religions is that of prayer. Despite diminishing physical health, persons of all religious beliefs tend to pray more during their senior years than at any other time in their lives

(Finley, 1989). Prayer is a practice with many faces. For a well elder, prayer may involve social interaction when engaged in during group worship services. For an ill or frail elder, private prayer or meditation can help alleviate feelings of loneliness or anxiety. For the confused or cognitively impaired older adult, traditional prayers learned in one's youth can sometimes be remembered and provide comfort. This is reflected in the comments of a chaplain with over seven years of experience in ministering to nursing home residents. In justifying the inclusion of confused elders in religious rites, the chaplain asserted:

> Even patients who are pretty much out of contact, they are
> still able to make the sign of the cross; they are still able to
> say prayers they learned when they were three or four years
> old. It [religion] is one of the things that goes last, as far as
> the memory is concerned; well, at least some basic tenets
> that they hang on to because they were so deeply ingrained.
> (O'Brien, 1989, p. 144)

Establishing a schedule for times of prayer during the day can be helpful for the newly retired person who may be somewhat "at loose ends"; the person can look forward to this time "not as a duty but as a time of joy and relaxation" (Coupland, 1985, p. 44). Some comforting Psalms that an elder might pray are Psalm 23, 'The Lord is my shepherd"; Psalm 25, Prayer for guidance; Psalm 34, God as protector; Psalm 62, Trust in God; Psalm 71, Prayer in old age; and Psalm 121, God's support in trials (Hynes, 1989, p. 49).

Spirituality and Physical Diminishment

When an elder's physical capacities are no longer functional at the level an individual may wish, a sense of inner comfort and peace may still be derived from spiritual beliefs and behaviors. Spiritual and religious practices such as meditation or silent prayer, or having a loving attitude toward others, may be part of a life plan even for the older old person afflicted with a multiplicity of physical deficits.

A nursing diagnosis of alteration in spiritual well-being or spiritual distress in an ill elder may be related to the individual's anger or frustration over an illness or disability. Chaplain Mary Brian Durkin, who ministers to patients on a rehabilitation unit, noted that a disabled patient's suffering was often associated with a negative attitude toward his or her condition (1992). For such a patient the provision of spiritual counseling and support can be a critical element in coping with illness and disability.

Spirituality and Cognitive Diminishment

Many older adults experience some degree of cognitive impairment as they progress through the aging process. Rice, Beck, and Stevenson (1997) reported that approximately 75 percent of nursing home residents have some cognitive impairment (p. 29). The latter statistic was supported during the author's conduct of an exploratory case study of a 230-bed nursing home, labeled "Bethany Manor" (O'Brien, 1989). Because of the large number of Bethany Manor residents manifesting dementia symptoms, an attempt was made, through qualitative interview, to gain at least minimal understanding of their spiritual, physical, and emotional needs. Some hints as to a resident's spirituality did emerge in the data, for example, remarks about God, prayer, or attendance at church as a child. One woman commented: "When you look at the handicaps all the people here have, I say God's been good to me" (p. 39); another long-term resident asserted: "I have been brought up as a Christian and my belief is a great support to me now" (p. 47).

Spiritual Needs of the Older Adult

In the face of debilitating or terminal illness, specific spiritual needs for trust, hope, and forgiveness most frequently manifest in an older adult. Related to these needs is the desire for reminiscence, which may help the elder to put present anxieties into the perspective of an entire lifetime.

Trust

Trust, a concept related to a sense of security in one's future, can be greatly tested during the later stages of the aging process. Fear of the unknown associated not only with death and the dying process but also with the concept of an afterlife poses a great threat to trust in the older adult. The religious elder who has lived according to the tenets of his or her tradition may more easily maintain trust by reflecting on the rewards identified for the faithful. An older adult who does not subscribe to any particular religious belief system will need to draw on personal philosophical beliefs about the meaning of life and one's own contribution to society for support.

Hope

Hope, or the expectation of a positive outcome in the future, is closely linked to trust, especially for the elder from a religious background. Hope is strengthened by an older adult's adherence to strong religious and moral values. Hope may be more difficult for an ill elder who no longer feels in control of his or her life or future activities. Hope engenders in an elder the spirit to find meaning and joy in life and to maintain a positive sense of self-worth amidst diminishing physical and psychological capacities.

Forgiveness

Perhaps the most frequently identified spiritual need for the older adult, especially in the face of serious or terminal illness, is the desire to give and to receive forgiveness. It is rare to find any person, especially one who has lived to elder years, who is not able to acknowledge some attitude or behavior for which he or she would wish forgiveness. The individual from whom the elder desires forgiveness may not be aware of the elder's need; the concern may totally reside in the heart and conscience of the one seeking forgiveness. The other important dimension of the concept relates to an older person's need to extend forgiveness to a person who in the elder's perception has done harm. To give and receive forgiveness are tasks not easily accomplished. It is important to remember, that desiring to forgive or accept forgiveness does not erase the memories; what forgiveness may accomplish is to "humanize" and incorporate a memory into an elder's current "self-understanding" (Maitland, 1991, p. 160). Healing occurs as the forgiving or forgiven elder reframes his or her self-image and is able to make peace with the past (Bozarth, 1995).

Reminiscence

Another need for the older adult, and one closely linked to giving or receiving forgiveness, is the need for reminiscence. As an individual reviews his or her life story, the need for forgiveness may emerge. There are also many other positive aspects to the act of reminiscence. First, an elder may be strengthened in dealing with present concerns and anxieties by remembering and reidentifying past coping skills used in dealing with stressful experiences. An elder may come to recognize that he or she has "endured beyond [the] ability to endure" (Seymour, 1995, p. 104). This can be a very beneficial memory in terms of facing the unknown future. The process of reviewing past life accomplishments can also serve to suggest what tasks an elder might still undertake, and what legacies can be left (Erikson, 1995, p. 14). In this way, reminiscence may serve as the catalyst for initiating a new career in later life or for helping the older adult to complete some partially finished tasks or activities. Additionally, an elder who reminisces as a social activity with family or friends can offer hard-earned wisdom as a gift to loved ones.

Spiritual Needs in Long-Term Care

Long-term health care for the elderly involves providing "comprehensive, continuous care for older adults in diverse settings" (Collins, Butler, Guelder, & Palmer, 1997, p. 59). These settings include the elder's home or the home of relatives, retirement communities, assisted care facilities, and skilled care nursing homes. The care populations consist of active elders with chronic illness, the homebound elderly, and elders in need of skilled nursing home care.

The Homebound Elder

Chronically ill elders who are homebound or nonmobile and living in assisted care facilities may have significant spiritual needs related to the physical and psychosocial sequelae of their conditions. The physical and emotional pain associated with being homebound requires a depth of faith and spirituality (Burghardt, 1991), as well as spiritual maturity, which Birren (1990) interpreted as the elder's ability to focus on transcendent spiritual values, while still appreciating religious experiences of the past (p. 42).

The Nursing Home Resident

The term *nursing home* is broadly understood as describing a facility that "provides twenty-four hour skilled nursing care at an intermediate [i.e., non-hospital] level" (Simmons & Peters, 1996,

p. 7). Presently almost 20 percent of older old adults (over 80) reside in nursing homes, and by the year 2030, the number is expected to triple (Koenig, 1994, p. 353). Data from an urban nursing home with approximately 230 residents revealed a population physical profile heavily laden with such diagnoses as arteriosclerotic heart disease, diabetes mellitus, hip fracture, osteoporosis, arthritis, Parkinson's disease, Alzheimer's disease, and senile dementia (O'Brien, 1989, pp. 22–23).

The multiplicity of health deficits experienced by current nursing home residents requires skill and ingenuity in care planning, including that of spiritual ministry. Malcolm (1987) believed that nurses must work at developing "creative spiritual care" for elderly nursing home residents; she suggested that although usual care plans place symptoms of dementia under a psychosocial need heading, these aspects of an elder's personality may also be "interwoven with the spiritual" (p. 25).

Some religious rituals appropriate for the responsive nursing home resident include Baptism (for one who has never experienced the sacrament earlier in life), Communion (according to the resident's religious tradition), Anointing of the Sick, and celebrations of religious feast days (Simmons & Peters, 1996, pp. 76–83). For the seriously physically or cognitively impaired resident, Simmons and Peters noted that these rituals may be adapted and modified to meet the elder's condition. Many nursing homes are formally affiliated with a particular religious denomination, so the worship services and rites of that tradition may be central to the home's activities; however, arrangements are generally made for religious ministry to residents of different traditions.

Three spiritual themes were derived from qualitative data elicited in the author's interviews with a nursing home group: faith in God and religious beliefs despite illness and disability, and acceptance of nursing home life; devotion, relating especially to private religious practices such as prayer and Scripture reading; and spiritual contentment, or a sense of peace in relation to where the elder is on his or her spiritual journey.

The Lord of the Nursing Home

Nursing homes are not places we look forward to visiting;
even the best of them, gifted with a spirit of
caring and compassion.
Nursing homes remind us of things we know,
but would rather forget:
We are grateful, Lord, for our years of
youth and strength; but we beg
You mightily to delay our years of age and fragility.

And yet we need not fear the nursing
home, Lord God of life, and death,
and glorious resurrection.
For You are there, Dear Lord,
as surely as You are in the cloistered monastery;
as surely as You are in the silent chapel;
as surely as You are in the majestic Cathedral.
You are there, O Lord of the Nursing Home:
in the gentle caring of a frail elder, who
bravely maneuvers her walker to visit
a bedridden comrade.

You are there, O Lord of the Nursing Home:
in the tender commitment of a faithful
daughter, who lovingly undertakes a frantic commute to
sit beside her senile mother.

You are there, O Lord of the Nursing Home:
in the kindness and compassion of a geriatric
nurse who caringly keeps watch at the bedside of a dying
patient.

You gift the nursing home with Your presence, O Lord;
and all who meet You there are blessed by Your love.

Contemporary elder adults are living longer and functioning better than ever before. Although obviously some physiological and psychosocial deficits accompany the aging process, a strong personal faith and participation in religious practices can greatly enhance an elder's quality of life. Chronically ill older adults living in a nursing care facility, as well as those living at home, may enjoy significant spiritual well-being in their later years. The aging adult may take comfort in the wisdom of Brother Roger of Taize who observed:

> *Every age has its own beauty. Why be afraid of physical decline when the years bring deeper insight and greater gentleness of action.*

(Cited in Finch, 1993, p. 23)

A Nurse's Prayer for a Compassionate Heart

> *When [Jesus] ... saw a great crowd; he had compassion for them, and cured their sick.*

MATTHEW 14:14

O God, who alone can grace my spirit with the gift of a compassionate heart, teach me to care. Help me to reach out to those who are in pain, to those who are lonely, to those who are afraid. Bless my nursing that I may become an instrument of Your tender understanding and Your love for those I serve. Let me be a vessel of compassion and caring in Your name. Amen.

References

Bianchi, E. C. (1995). *Aging as a spiritual journey*. New York: Cross-road.

Birren, J. E. (1990). Spiritual maturity in psychological development. In J. Seeber (Ed.), *Spiritual maturity in the later years* (pp. 41–53). New York: The Haworth Press.

Bozarth, A. R. (1995). *Lifelines: Threads of grace through seasons of change*. Kansas City, MO: Sheed & Ward.

Burghardt, W. J. (1991). Aging, suffering and dying: A Christian perspective. In L. S. Cahill & D. Mieth (Eds.), *Aging* (pp. 65–71). London: Conciliam.

Burt, D. X. (1992). *But when you are older: Reflections on coming of age*. Collegeville, MN: The Liturgical Press.

Collins, C. E., Butler, F. R., Guelder, S. H., & Palmer, M. H. (1997). Models for community-based long-term care for the elderly in a changing health system. *Nursing Outlook, 45*(2), 59–63.

Coupland, S. (1985). *Beginning to pray in old age*. Cambridge, MA: Cowley.

Durkin, M. B. (1992). A community of caring. *Health Progress, 73*(8), 48–53.

Erickson, R. M. (1995). *Late have I loved thee: Stories of religious conversion and commitment in later life*. New York: Paulist Press.

Finch, A. (Ed.). (1993). *Journey to the light: Spirituality as we mature*. New Rochelle, NY: New City Press.

Finley, J. (1989). *The treasured age: Spirituality for seniors*. New York: Alba House.

Fowler, J. W. (1981). *Stages of faith: The psychology of human development and the quest for meaning*. San Francisco: Harper.

Hynes, M. (1989). *The ministry to the aging*. Collegeville, MN: The Liturgical Press.

Koenig, H. G. (1994). *Aging and God: Spiritual pathways to mental health in midlife and later years*. New York: The Haworth Press.

Maitland, D. J. (1991). *Aging as counterculture: A vocation for the later years*. New York: The Pilgrim Press.

Malcolm, J. (1987). Creative spiritual care for the elderly. *Journal of Christian Nursing*, 4(1), 24–26.

O'Brien, M. E. (1989). *Anatomy of a nursing home: A new view of resident life*. Owings Mills, MD: National Health Publishing.

Peterson, V., & Potter, P. A. (1997). Spiritual health. In P. A. Potter & A. G. Perry (Eds.), *Fundamentals of nursing: Concepts, process and practice* (pp. 440–455). St. Louis, MO: C. V. Mosby.

Rice, V. H., Beck, C., & Stevenson, J. S. (1997). Ethical issues relative to autonomy and personal control in independent and cognitively impaired elders. *Nursing Outlook*, 45(1), 27–34.

Roen, O. T. (1997). Senior health. In J. H. Swanson & M. A. Nies (Eds.), *Community health nursing: Promoting the health of aggregates* (2nd ed., pp. 347–386). Philadelphia: W. B. Saunders.

Seymour, R. E. (1995). *Aging without apology: Living the senior years with integrity and faith*. Valley Forge, PA: Judson Press.

Simmons, H. C., & Peters, M. A. (1996). *With God's oldest friends: Pastoral visiting in the nursing home*. New York: Paulist Press.

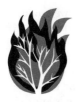

CHAPTER 9

Spiritual Care in Death and Bereavement

For everything there is a season, and a time for every matter under heaven; a time to be born and a time to die.

ECCLESIASTES 3:1-2

There Is a Time

Dear Father in heaven,
You have taught us that, for everything, there is a time:

"A time to be born and a time to die" (Ecclesiastes 3:2).
Teach us to embrace both the beginning and the end of life, as Your gifts.

"A time to mourn and a time to dance" (Ecclesiastes 3:4).
Grant us the understanding to honor You in our gifts; and the wisdom to bless You in their loss.

"A time to seek and a time to lose" (Ecclesiastes 3:6).
Help us to know when to rejoice in our good health; and when to glory in our infirmity.

"A time to keep silence and a time to speak"
(Ecclesiastes 3:7).

Grace us with the ability to accept the things we cannot change; and the courage to advocate for the things we can influence.

"A time for war and a time for peace" (Ecclesiastes 3:8). Counsel us to fight valiantly against illness and disability; but endow us with acceptance when the battle is lost.

Help us, Dearest Lord, to remember that, in all things, there is a time; a time that is not ours, a time that, blessedly, is Yours.

From a theological perspective, death is conceptualized as "the final point of a human person's individual history . . . the decisive act of human freedom in which the person can either accept or reject the mystery of God and thereby put the final seal on his or her personal history and destiny" (Hayes, 1993, pp. 272–273). The spiritual understanding of death is undergirded by an individual's religious belief, that is, faith tradition. In Judaism attitudes toward death vary both within and among specific traditions: Orthodox, Conservative, Reform, and Reconstructionist. In general, however, Judaism places great value on life as God's gift; there may be uncertainty about the existence of an afterlife (Neuberger, 1994). Christian spirituality views death and dying in terms of the Gospel message of Jesus. Jesus' death provides a model for His followers who accept their sufferings in hope of the eternal reward He promised. For Jesus, death was not an ending but the beginning of eternal life.

The Spirituality of Death and Dying

How a person dies can reveal a great deal about how he or she lived. So also, the spirituality manifested in death and in the dying process reflects the personal spirituality of the dying person. For a dying individual who adheres to the tenets of a religious denomination that professes belief in an afterlife, the dying process can represent a joyful transition to a better state, a place where the good acts of one's life are rewarded and sins are absolved. For the person who believes that existence of both body and spirit cease with physical death, the dying process may represent a fearful experience, especially if the individual has not fulfilled desired life goals and ambitions. Spiritual care will need to be carefully planned so as to be relevant to the prevailing spiritual and religious beliefs of the dying patient and his or her family. Many deaths occur in the hospital, nursing home, or hospice setting. With changes in the contemporary health care system, however, more and more terminally ill individuals will die at home. Thus, the provision of spiritual support for patient and family may fall to the home health care or parish nurse, as well as to hospital, hospice, or nursing home nursing staff.

Spiritual Needs in the Dying Process

The dying process is unique to each person; a multiplicity of demographic, physical, psychosocial, and spiritual values may influence and mediate the experience. Such factors as age, gender, marital status, religious tradition, socioeconomic status, diagnosis, coping skills, social support, and spiritual belief, especially as related to the meaning of life and death, can influence one's management of the dying process. Despite the uniqueness of the individual, however, some universal needs are identified for most dying persons. These include the need for relief from loneliness and isolation, the need to feel useful, the need to express anger, the need for comfort in anxiety and fear, and the need to alleviate depression and find meaning in the experience (Kemp, 1995, pp. 11–16). Kenneth Doka (1993b) posited three broadly circumscribed spiritual goals of the dying person: "(1) to identify the meaning of one's life, (2) to die appropriately, and (3) to find hope that extends beyond the grave" (p. 146). Other spiritual needs of the dying person identified in the nursing literature include the need for forgiveness and love (Conrad, 1985), for self-acceptance, and for positive relationships with others, including, for some, relationship with God or a deity (Highfield, 1992).

Although the physical and psychosocial needs of the dying may be more readily identified by overt emotional or physical symptoms, spiritual needs can be more difficult to assess. Because one's spiritual and religious beliefs are personal, symptoms of spiritual distress may not be openly displayed and thus may be neglected in the planning of care for a dying patient (Charlton, 1992). Such lack of attention to spiritual needs is not acceptable, however, for nurses attempting to provide holistic care during the dying process (Stepnick & Perry, 1992).

Tim, a 37-year-old terminal cancer patient, explained the importance of resolving spiritual issues prior to his impending death: "I guess it's like they say about 'no atheists in fox holes.' Well I'm in more than a foxhole. I need to get things together with myself and God before I go. I'm praying, and a pastor's been coming by to see me. I guess you don't think about all this until it gets near the end, but it's time now; it's definitely time."

Spiritual Care in Death and Dying

Dying patients and their families cope with impending death in a variety of ways, depending on such factors as the age of the patient, the severity of the illness, the patient's religious beliefs, and cultural norms and values. One of the most frequently observed dilemmas is the fluctuation between acceptance and denial of the immediacy of death. Helping dying patients and families to manage the tension between these two attitudes is a key role of the spiritual caregiver (Joesten, 1992). Some broad areas of spiritual nursing care for dying persons include assisting the patient to find meaning in life, hope, a relationship to God, forgiveness or acceptance, and transcendence (Kemp, 1995, p. 45). Five specific spiritual interventions for dying patients that fall within the purview of the nurse are praying, facilitating the presence of loved ones, allowing the dying person time to share, assisting in the completion of unfinished tasks, and assuring that the dying person has been given "permission" to die (Olson, 1997, p. 133). Nurses caring for dying patients should also attempt to identify the presence of spiritual pain, which may be manifested in terms of "the past (painful memories, regret, failure, guilt); the present (isolation, unfairness, anger); the future (fear, hopelessness)" (Eisdon, 1995, p. 641).

Religious Practices in Death and Dying

For a dying person, religious practices can provide an important dimension of spiritual support and comfort. Even if an individual has become alienated from a religious denomination or church, a terminal illness may be the catalyst for return to the practice of one's faith. This was clearly reflected in the comments of a 47-year-old male patient in the advanced stages of cancer: "I hadn't gone to my church for years; I don't know why. I just stopped going. But lately I've started up again, and I've been reading the Bible. When I die I want to have a church burial and be buried in a Christian cemetery; that's a big thing with my family."

Although the nurse caring for dying patients cannot be knowledgeable about the death-related beliefs and practices of all religious faiths, some familiarity with those of the major Western and Eastern traditions may provide a starting point for the provision of spiritual support. Having some idea of the theological positions and religious practices of different groups may assist the nurse in developing a relationship with a dying person and an empathetic and caring attitude (Head, 1994, p. 310).

The Western Tradition: Judaism, Christianity, and Islam

Judaism

Attitudes toward death for the Jewish patient may vary according to identification with a particular subgroup of Judaism: Orthodox, Conservative, Reform, or Reconstructionist. A Jewish person's approach to the dying process will also be influenced by his or her belief or nonbelief in the existence of an afterlife. Some Jews, especially those of the Orthodox tradition, do not subscribe to the concept of eternal life; they may, however, believe that faithful Jews will be resurrected when the Messiah comes. Some believe that one's good deeds in this life live on in the memories of family and friends. In Judaism, life is highly valued as a gift of God; all efforts to continue a productive life are supported. Thus, facing death may represent an ending of something precious. As Rabbi Julia Neuberger (1994) explained, "It is not so much uncertainty about the afterlife which causes a problem, but the emphasis put on the here and now" (p. 13).

A Jewish person who is dying, especially an Orthodox Jew, will generally receive visits from friends and synagogue members, because the duty to visit the sick is considered a *mitzvah* or good deed in Judaism. Some contemporary synagogues have established formalized groups called *Bikkur Cholim* societies, whose express purpose is to visit and minister to those who are ill; *Bikkur Cholim* members receive training from their synagogues in how to work with the sick. These individuals may also be present at a Jewish person's death and will offer prayers or readings from the Psalms, if desired by the patient or family.

After death occurs, synagogue members from the Jewish Burial Society may come to prepare the body of an Orthodox patient; no action should be taken by hospital or hospice personnel until it is determined whether this will occur. It is also customary that, after death, a Jewish person be buried within 24 hours; an exception may be made for the Sabbath. The formal ritual prayer of mourning, the *kaddish*, may be recited by a rabbi or family member; cremation and autopsy are avoided. After the burial has taken place, the important task of mourning is initiated. This involves friends and relatives of the deceased visiting at the family's home, or sitting *shiva* for the next seven days. This mourning period provides the grieving family with the support and care of those close to them and to the deceased person during the time immediately following death. Following *shiva*, 30 days of mourning, *sh-loshim*, continues; during this time the family may resume usual activities but avoids formal entertainment (Grollman, 1993).

Christianity

Three major subgroups within the Christian tradition are the Eastern Orthodox Churches, Roman Catholicism, and Protestantism; in addition, a number of other faith groups are identified as followers of Christ. Virtually all Christian traditions believe in eternal life, as promised in the Gospel message of Jesus. Thus, for the devout Christian, although the dying process can raise anxieties in terms of possible pain and suffering, death itself is viewed as a positive transition to a life with God and to one's eternal reward. Protestantism, which relies on the concept of salvation, trusts that faith will bring the believer into a better world (Klass, 1993). Older adult Christians sometimes express a desire for God to come and "take them home."

As death approaches, the majority of Christian patients and their families welcome a visit from a priest or minister; the pastoral visitor may be from the family's church or can be a hospital or hospice chaplain. These ministers will generally pray and read a Scripture passage with the dying person and their family. Eastern Orthodox Christians, Roman Catholics, and some Episcopalians may request an anointing or the "Sacrament of the Sick" prior to death; they may also wish to make a confession of sins and receive the sacraments of Penance and of Holy Eucharist (Holy Communion). A priest or family member may cross the arms of the Eastern Orthodox patient after death, situating the fingers to represent a cross.

After death occurs, most Christians will have a period of "viewing" of the body, sometimes called a "wake"; this ritual, which provides the opportunity for friends and family to call, takes place from one to three days after the death, in either the family home or a funeral home. A priest or minister may offer prayers periodically during the viewing. Christian burial services vary according to denomination. Eastern Orthodox, Roman Catholic, and some Episcopalian (Anglo-Catholic) Christians attend a funeral Mass of Requiem for the deceased prior to interment in a church cemetery. Although Mass is still the norm for the Catholic funeral, emphasis is now placed on life rather than death, and the central theme is resurrection; the priest celebrant wears white rather than black vestments. This changed focus, from grieving the death to hope in God's love and trust in the resurrection, indicates "a more healthy biblicism and pastoral practice" (Miller, 1993, p. 42). Other Christians participate in funeral or memorial services of their denominations; some families prefer a private service conducted by a minister in the home. The latter may be desired if cremation is chosen and no formal trip to the cemetery is planned.

Islam

The devout Muslim, like the Christian, views death as representing a spiritual transition to eternal life with Allah (Renard, 1993). Although a terminally ill Muslim may fear the dying process related to possible suffering, the concept of death itself is accepted as the will of Allah. Thus, excessive grieving of death by a Muslim may be considered inappropriate and represent a contradiction of Allah's plan. The death of a loved one should be viewed as only a temporary loss (Neuberger, 1994, p. 36). Islam, like Christianity, holds a belief in "resurrection of the body, final judgement and assignment to heaven or hell" (Kemp, 1995, p. 58).

As death approaches, family members or a Muslim minister, an imam, may read a passage from the Holy Qur'an to comfort the patient and family. The dying Muslim may wish to face Mecca, in the East, and ask forgiveness of Allah for sins. After death occurs, members of the family frequently wish to prepare the body through ritual washing and wrapping in a white cloth. After the body is prepared, the deceased may be laid out in a position facing Mecca.

Burial rites for a Muslim patient can vary, but generally interment takes place in a Muslim cemetery 24 hours after death.

The Eastern Tradition: Hinduism, Buddhism, and Confucianism

Hinduism

Hinduism, as described in Chapter 3, consists of a number of related Indian religious traditions, all of which are centuries old. Although a pantheon of lesser gods is associated with Hinduism, as demonstrated in Indian temples and holy places, most devout Hindus believe in the existence of one supreme being or deity. The many less powerful gods and goddesses are considered to be forms or derivatives of the one deity, with power and interest in specific areas of one's life.

The concept of reincarnation or rebirth influences the dying Hindu's attitude toward death; death itself is viewed as union with God. How one has lived in this world is influential in how one might return in the next life; this concept is referred to as karma.

Hindu patients often prefer to die at home where they can be more certain of the presence of a priest (Green, 1989a). A Brahmin priest, who performs the death rites, may tie a string or cord around the dying person's neck or wrist which should not be removed; prayers are also chanted by the priest. Following a Hindu's death, the funeral is usually carried out within 24 hours, and cremation is the traditional ritual.

Buddhism

Buddhism, founded by Gautama Siddhartha, differs from most other major religious traditions in that the Buddhist does not accept the existence of God or of a Supreme Being; Buddhists do however, acknowledge the presence of a multiplicity of individual gods who are involved and interested in the lives of the Buddhist. Devout Buddhists live according to the "eightfold path" of right belief, right intent, right speech, right conduct, right endeavor, right mindfulness, right effort, and right meditation (Kemp, 1995, p. 60). The ultimate goal of the Buddhist is to reach the interior state of Nirvana or inner peace and happiness; this is achieved after having lived according to the eightfold path.

The Buddhist's attitude toward death is also influenced by belief in the concept of rebirth; death is accepted as a transition and as part of the cycle of life. A Buddhist monk may chant prayers at the death of a devout Buddhist in order to provide peace of mind at the point of death (Green, 1989b). An important dimension of the dying process for a Buddhist is to remain conscious in order to be able to think right and wholesome thoughts (Kemp, 1995). The deceased is generally cremated after death.

Confucianism

Confucianism is the tradition founded by the ancient Chinese scholar and philosopher, Confucius. Confucianism places great emphasis on respecting the memories and the contributions of one's ancestors. Elaborate death and burial rituals allow the bereaved to formally express grief and bring "continuity with the past and with tradition" (Ryan, 1993, p. 85). Ryan (1993) reported that in the Confucian tradition a person is taught to live life in such a way that after death good memories of the deceased may be honored (p. 86). The fate of the deceased in an afterlife depends on the quality of his or her natural life; it is also important that the deceased be properly honored by relatives after death. This relates to a strong belief in a "continuity of life after death" (Neuberger, 1994, p. 48).

The Confucianist's funeral may be an elaborate ritual, its complexity reflecting the status of the deceased. A carefully crafted coffin may be purchased by the family prior to death so that the dying person will know that he or she will be well honored at the burial rites.

Spiritual Care in Bereavement

The body of literature dealing with the post-death period includes the terms *bereavement*, *grief*, and *mourning*; these are sometimes used interchangeably, all being understood as describing the physical and psychosocial experience of loss following the death of a loved one. Historically, the study of the bereavement experience, including the aspects of grief and mourning, began with the work of Eric Lindemann in 1944. His classic study of 101 bereaved survivors of Boston's "Coconut Grove" fire provided the benchmark for our contemporary understanding of the grieving process. Lindemann described the acute reaction to the death of a loved one as including such somatic responses as "a feeling of tightness in the throat; choking with shortness of breath; need for sighing; an empty feeling in the abdomen; lack of muscular power; and an intense subjective distress described as tension or mental pain" (p. 141). Manifestations of an uncomplicated grief reaction are generally divided into four categories: physical, cognitive, emotional, and behavioral. Some of these as described by Worden (1982) include physical reactions such as stomach emptiness, shortness of breath, tightness in chest and throat, and fatigue; cognitive reactions of disbelief and mental confusion; emotional responses of sadness, guilt, anger, loneliness, numbness, and yearning for the deceased; and behavioral disruptions such as insomnia, loss of appetite, social isolation, crying, and restlessness (pp. 20–23).

Bereaved persons need and will often accept spiritual support from the family's pastoral care provider, rabbi, minister, priest, or, in some cases, a nurse if he or she is skilled in bereavement counseling and support. Other significant persons who may provide spiritual support for the bereaved are church or faith group members who also understand the grieving person's or family's spiritual and theological perspective on the loss. Whether spiritual care is provided by the pastor, nurse, or church member, intervention should focus on supporting two major tasks of the bereaved individual: letting go of the deceased person and becoming reinvested in current life activities. The spiritual caregiver's challenge in grief and bereavement is to balance the activities of strengthening and disputing; the caregiver must "know when to comfort and support and when to challenge and confront" (Joesten, 1992, p. 144). Joesten observed that an important dimension of spiritual intervention for bereaved persons is the presence of a caring other who is willing to be there and share in the grief and the pain (p. 145); he asserted that the spiritual caregiver assists the bereaved most by being someone who offers hope and honesty amidst the darkness of the experience (p. 148).

Although normal grief encompasses many physical and psychosocial sequelae with which the bereaved must cope, complicated or dysfunctional grief may present even more suffering. Dysfunctional grief has many descriptions; it is generally believed to occur when the usual tasks of the grieving process are thwarted or blocked. Some factors that might be associated with a dysfunctional grief reaction are an unhealthy relationship between the deceased and the bereaved, poor coping skills on the part of the mourner, a lack of material and social support in the bereavement experience, and inadequate mental or physical health of the bereaved (Kemp, 1995, p. 77).

A more recently identified dysfunctional type of response to loss has been labeled "disenfranchised grief." Disenfranchised grief is defined as "the grief that persons experience when they incur a loss that is not, or cannot be openly acknowledged, publicly mourned, or socially supported" (Doka, 1989, p. 4). Doka posited that a survivor may be disenfranchised for three reasons: "the relationship is not recognized," for example, in the case of a child of an unwed mother who is unable to mourn a nonacknowledged father; "the loss is not recognized," such as the loss of a child to abortion or miscarriage; and "the griever is not recognized," as in the case of a mentally retarded or disabled survivor (pp. 5–7). In disenfranchised grief, as the tasks of grieving must be carried out privately without the support of family and friends, the bereaved person can be forced into a state of silent unresolved grief that may last for many years. Pastoral counselor Dale Kuhn (1989) pointed out that despite a negative or unsatisfactory experience with a church or faith group, a bereaved person experiencing disenfranchised grief may still continue to seek support from God; in this situation the individual spiritual caregiver may play an important role as a counseling and listening presence in the silent grieving process (p. 247).

Personal spirituality and religiosity or religious practice are important mediating variables in coping with death and bereavement. Dying persons' and their families' spiritual and religious beliefs about such concepts as the meaning of life and death, the existence of an afterlife, and the purpose of suffering can influence profoundly how the dying process is experienced. The nurse, sensitive to the spiritual and religious beliefs of a dying patient and his or her family, may be able to provide therapeutic spiritual support and intervention that will mediate the pain associated with the death and bereavement experiences.

A Nurse's Prayer "To Proclaim the Kingdom"

> Dear Lord Jesus, You call me, and you "send"
> me (Luke 9:1) to "proclaim the
> kingdom . . . and to heal" the sick.
> > (Luke 9:2)

> You ask me to "take nothing" for the "journey"; neither
> walking stick . . . nor food, nor money."
> > (Luke 9:3)

This is not a very comforting message, Dear Lord: no
food, not even a little money in case I get hungry?

You know I'll be taken care of, My Lord and my God,
for your faith is infinite; but my hope is so fragile.

What if I don't have the strength,
or the courage, or the talent to heal the sick and
proclaim the kingdom? These are heavy mandates, Lord
Jesus. You yourself, appointed disciples to carry them out

But, then, that's the heart of this call, isn't it, Dear Lord?

It's not my mission to proclaim the gospel and heal the
sick, but Yours!

It's not my task to worry about the talent and the
courage, and the strength, but Yours!

It's not my grace that makes me a minister of the gospel,
but Yours!

Teach me to trust.

References

Charlton, R. G. (1992). Spiritual need of the dying and bereaved:
Views from the United Kingdom and New Zealand. *Journal of
Palliative Care*, 8(4), 38–40.

Conrad, N. L. (1985). Spiritual support for the dying. *Nursing Clinics
of North America*, 20(2), 415–426.

Doka, K. J. (1989). *Disenfranchised grief: Recognizing hidden sorrow*.
Lexington, MA: Lexington Books.

Doka, K.J. (1993). The spiritual needs of the dying. In K.J. Doka
(Ed.), *Death and spirituality* (pp. 143–150). Amityville, NY:
Beywood.

Eisdon, R. (1995). Spiritual pain in dying people: The nurse's role. *Professional Nurse*, 10(10), 641–643.

Green, J. (1989a). Death with dignity: Hinduism. *Nursing Times*, 85(6), 50–51.

Green, J. (1989b). Death with dignity: Buddhism. *Nursing Times*, 85(9), 40–41.

Grollman, E. A. (1993). Death in Jewish thought. In K. J. Doka (Ed.), *Death and spirituality* (pp. 21–32). Amityville, NY: Baywood.

Hayes, Z. (1993). Death. In J. A. Komonchak, M. Collins, & D. A. Lane (Eds.), *The new dictionary of theology*. Collegeville, MN: The Liturgical Press.

Head, D. (1994). Religious approaches to dying. In I. B. Corless, B. B. Germino, & M. Pittman (Eds.), *Dying, death and bereavement: Theoretical perspectives and other ways of knowing*. Boston: Jones and Bartlett.

Highfield, M.F. (1992). Spiritual health of oncology patients: Nurse and patient perspectives. *Cancer Nursing*, 15(1), 1–8.

Highfield, M. E., Taylor, E. J., & Amenta, M. O. (2000). Preparation to care: The spiritual care education of oncology and hospice nurses. *Journal of Hospice and Palliative Nursing*, 2(2), 53–63.

Joesten, L. B. (1992). The voices of the dying and the bereaved: A bridge between loss and growth. In L. E. Holst (Ed.), *Hospital ministry: The role of the chaplain today* (pp. 139-150). New York: Crossroad.

Kemp, C. (1995). *Terminal illness: A guide to nursing care*. Philadelphia: J. B. Lippincott.

Klass, D. (1993). Spirituality, Protestantism and death. In K. J. Doka (Ed.), *Death and spirituality* (pp. 51–74). Amityville, NY: Baywood.

Kuhn, D. (1989). A pastoral counselor looks at silence as a factor in disenfranchised grief. In K. J. Doka (Ed.), *Disenfranchised grief: Recognizing hidden sorrow* (pp. 241–256). Lexington, MA: Lexington Books.

Lindemann, E. (1944). Symptomatology and management of acute grief. *American Journal of Psychiatry*, 101(1), 141–148.

Miller, E. J. (1993). A Roman Catholic view of death. In K. J. Doka (Ed.), *Death and spirituality* (pp. 33–50). Amityville, NY: Baywood.

Neuberger, J. (1994). *Caring for dying people of different faiths* (2nd ed.). St. Louis, MO: C. V. Mosby.

Olson, M. (1997). *Healing the dying*. New York: Delmar.

Renard, J. (1993). Islamic spirituality. In M. Downey (Ed.), *The new dictionary of Catholic spirituality* (pp. 555–559). Collegeville, MN: The Liturgical Press.

Ryan, D. (1993). Death: Eastern perspectives. In K. J. Doka (Ed.), *Death and spirituality* (pp. 75–92). Amityville, NY: Baywood.

Stepnick, A., & Perry, T. (1992). Preventing spiritual distress in the dying client. *Journal of Psychosocial Nursing*, 30(1), 17–24.

Worden, J. W. (1982). *Grief counseling and grief therapy: A handbook for the mental health practitioner*. New York: Springer.

CHAPTER 10

Parish Nursing: Healthcare Ministry Within the Church

Jesus called the twelve . . . and he sent them out to proclaim the kingdom of God and to heal.

LUKE 9:1

Lord, When Did I Care for You? A Parish Nurse's Meditation

Dear Lord,
"I beg your help," You said to me; "so many
of my children are in need.
They're sick, and they're anxious and they're lonely; and
there's no one to care for them.
The harvest is plentiful but the laborers are few
(Luke 10:2).
Won't you become one of my laborers?; and care for Me?"
"I don't have time, right now," Dear Lord, I answered
at first.
"Couldn't you ask someone else? I have so much 'busi-
ness' to attend to,"
(Matthew 22:5).
And, needing another defense, I added: "All of Your
commandments 'I have kept since my youth';
(Mark 10:20).

Isn't that enough?"
But then, You looked at me, Lord, with that look; the
one that said you 'loved me'; and it rent my heart.
"Come follow me."

(Mark 10:21)

You whispered gently, and I was helpless.
And so, I followed You, Dearest Lord;
I became Your laborer.
I have cared for Your children: those who
were sick, and those who were anxious,
and those who were lonely, but when,
my Lord and my God, did I care for You?
Jesus replied: "When you fed a frail parishioner
so the family could rest, you gave Me food.
"When you got a drink of water for a parishioner's sick
child, you gave Me drink.
"When you invited a new parishioner to tell you her
needs, you welcomed Me.
"When you brought a warm sweater to a wheelchair-
bound parishioner, you clothed Me.
"When you counseled a parishioner diagnosed with
cancer, you cared for Me."
And,
"When you prayed with a parishioner
confined to a nursing home, you visited Me.
"In all of your ministries to these, my 'little ones,'
Dear parish nurse," the Lord replied: "You cared for Me."
"And so," He added: "I shall, one day have another
invitation for you, which I will issue with great joy":
"Come, you that are blessed by my Father.
Inherit the kingdom prepared for you from the
foundation of the world."

(Matthew 25:34).

Parish Nursing Defined

Essentially, the philosophy of parish nursing is grounded in the relationship between spirituality or faith beliefs and the conduct of caring for the sick. This might be described best in the following paradigm of "Beatitudes for Parish Nurses," which combines the Scriptural beatitudes identified by Jesus in His Sermon on the Mount (Matthew 5:3–10) with the primary roles identified for contemporary parish nurses: health counselor, health educator (health promoter), health referral agent, health advocate, health visitor, integrator of faith and health, coordinator of support and volunteer groups.

Beatitudes for Parish Nurses

> Blessed are parish nurses who care for the poor,
>   for theirs is the kingdom of heaven.
> Blessed are parish nurses who mourn for parishioners
>   lost, for they will be comforted.
> Blessed are parish nurses who visit the isolated and the
>   elderly, for they will inherit the land.
> Blessed are parish nurses who advocate for marginalized
>   clients, for they will be satisfied.
> Blessed are parish nurses who minister to those in pain
>   and suffering, for they will be shown mercy.
> Blessed are parish nurses who bring peace to patients
>   who are anxious and afraid, for they will be called
>   children of God.
> Blessed are parish nurses who suffer misunderstanding
>   for the sake of their ministry, for they will see God.
> Blessed are parish nurses who comfort and care in the
>   Lord's Name, for their reward will be great in heaven.

The philosophy of parish nursing has been described as the guiding principle to "promote the health of a faith community by working with the pastor and staff to integrate theological, sociological and physiological perspectives of health and healing into the word, sacrament and service of the congregation" (Lovinus, 1996, p. 7). The parish nurse serves as "a role model for the relationship between one's faith and health" (Solari-Twadell & Westberg, 1991, p. 24).

The parish nurse is considered by most parish nurse educators to be a registered nurse with well-developed clinical and interpersonal skills, a strong personal religious faith, and a desire or felt call to serve the needs of a parish or faith community. A parish nursing philosophy builds on the existing philosophy of caring and commitment already espoused by the nurse as a professional ethic. One parish nurse described her ministry as a vocation: "Nursing in a faith community is a calling, an absolute caring for people and a deep sense of personal faith" (Palmer, 2001, p. 17). Parish nurses are generally noted for their roles as educators and health promoters within a congregation. "They provide information on healthy life styles and ways to prevent illness" (Dunkle, 2000, p. 316); they also, however, tend to patients' "psychosocial and spiritual needs" (p. 316).

Scope and Standards of Parish Nursing Practice

Between 1996 and 1998, a document identifying the scope and standards of parish nursing practice was developed by the Practice and Education Committee of the Health Ministries Association (HMA). The HMA is a professional organization that represents parish nurses and other health ministers. The scope and standards document was acknowledged by the American Nurses Association, Congress of Nursing Practice, in Spring 1998. The introduction to the document states that "Parish nursing promotes health and healing within faith communities" (Scope and Standards of Parish Nursing Practice, 1998, p. 1).

The purpose of the scope and standards document is to "describe the evolving specialty of parish nursing and to provide parish nurses, the nursing profession, and other health care providers, employers, insurers, and their clients with the unique scope and competent standards of care and professional performance expected of a parish nurse" (1998, p. 3). The parish nurse scope and standards are based on the ANA's 1991 Standards of Clinical Nursing Practice. The definition of parish nurse, as articulated formally in the scope and standards of practice is: "The most common title given to a registered professional nurse who serves as a member of the ministry staff of a faith community to promote health as wholeness of the faith community, its family and individual members, and the community it serves through the independent practice of nursing as defined by the nurse practice act in the jurisdiction in which he or she practices and the standards of practice set forth in this document" (1998, p. 7).

Some of the parish nurse's roles, as identified in the scope and standards of practice include: collecting client health data (health assessment); diagnosing, based on the data; identifying desired health outcomes; health care and promotion planning; implementing interventions; and evaluating client responses (1998, pp. 9–14).

The History of Parish Nursing

The contemporary concept of parish nursing is attributed to Lutheran pastor Granger Westberg, as an outgrowth of his holistic health center project of the mid-1980s (Westburg, 1990). Although Pastor Westberg is appropriately acknowledged as the founder of the current parish nursing movement in the United States, one should also recognize the health care activities of the early Christian Church, as well as the European models of parish nursing, such as the 19th century German Christian Deaconesses, the *Gemeindeschwestern* (Zerson, 1994, p. 20). The earliest deacons and deaconesses of the fledgling Christian community, established immediately after the death of Christ, considered care of the sick in their homes to be one of the primary ministries of the Church. Following those early centuries and throughout the Middle Ages, men and women felt their calling to minister to the ill and the infirm to be a vocation from God.

The International Parish Nurse Resource Center (IPNRC) was created in 1986, under the aegis of Advocate Lutheran General Hospital. Together with a committee of nurse consultants from across the country, the staff of the IPNRC developed a model curriculum for parish nursing education. The IPNRC also began to sponsor annual Westberg Symposiums to provide a forum for parish nurses from across the country to come together to discuss the emerging subfield and its practice. In an October 2001 letter addressed to the "Friends of the International Parish Nurse Resource Center," however, it was announced that the IPNRC would no longer be an agency of Advocate Health Care, the umbrella organization providing support for this parish nursing education effort. As of December 31, 2002, sponsorship of the IPNRC was transferred to Deaconess Parish Health Ministries, St. Louis, Missouri. The International Parish Nurse Resource center under the aegis of Deaconess Parish Health Ministries continues to support the Parish Nurse curriculum, as well as other activities initiated by the IPNRC in Illinois.

Another parish nursing association, this one a volunteer membership group labeled the Health Ministries Association (HMA), was derived from the emerging parish nursing interest of the '70s and '80s. The HMA, author of the "Scope and Standards of Nursing Practice," is an association for those who serve in health ministry. The group "serves as the professional specialty organization for parish nurses and as such has been accepted by the American Nurses Association for membership in the Nursing Organization Liaison Forum (NOLF)" (FAQ about HMA & Parish Nursing, 2001, p. 1).

Parish Nursing Education

Related to the emerging models of parish nursing are a variety of educational programs that prepare one for the field of parish nursing. These educational offerings range from weekend or week-long continuing education unit (CEU) programs, which may award from three to six CEUs, to academic courses in parish nursing, ranging from three to six credits for the overall program. There are also several post-baccalaureate and graduate programs that focus on the topic of nursing in a faith community. These programs are sponsored primarily by health care institutions, colleges and universities, seminaries, or other church-related associations. In some instances, community interfaith groups of churches have collaboratively put together parish nurse education programs to prepare nurses to serve in their various faith communities. The multiplicity of parish nurse preparation programs are, as noted earlier, conducted in a variety of ways; some of these include "one day to week long orientations, continuing education workshops, seminars, distance learning, and ongoing coursework over weeks and months, as well as credit-bearing coursework in BSN, MSN and M.Div. programs offered over the course of a semester or, for some, over several years" (McDermott, Solari-Twadell, & Matheus, 1999, p. 271).

Three examples of contemporary parish nurse programs are:

- A week-long continuing education program, sponsored by a Christian nursing group, following which the participants are awarded three CEUs and are "commissioned" as parish nurses. Requirements for the course include having a state nursing license, some clinical nursing experience, and the desire to work with a faith community.

- A parish nurse preparation program, sponsored by a college and awarding the participants three CEUs, which holds classes on six alternating Saturdays. This program requires that the RNs have at least three years experience and be partnered with a faith community. The course ends with a "dedication ceremony".

- A university-affiliated program that covers nine days and awards the participants 5.4 CEUs. As well as including the usual topics described below, this longer program includes participation in several interfaith services and provides student on-site observations and clinical experiences with parish nurses in the community.

Some basic components of most contemporary parish nursing programs include such topics as: a theology of health and healing; the nurse's role in spiritual care; history, philosophy, and models of parish nursing; ethical issues in parish nursing; assessment of the individual, the family, and the congregation; documentation and accountability; the functions of the parish nurse, such as health counseling, health education, health referral, co-ordination of volunteers and support groups, patient advocacy, and integration of faith and health; working with a congregation; health promotion; dealing with grief and loss; and legal considerations in the conduct of parish nursing. Some programs also include classes focusing on such activities as prayer and worship leadership, research, grant writing, service among underprivileged people, and working with a ministerial team.

The Ministry of Parish Nursing

Although nurses from a variety of religious denominations are currently engaged in parish nursing, it is the nurse's personal spirituality and spiritual vocation to serve the ill that inspire and support the ministry. For Christian nurses, Jesus' blessing, related by the evangelist Matthew "I was ill and you cared for me" (25:36) provides both the catalyst and the reward for their caring for the sick within a faith community. Most parish nurses, many of whom serve on a volunteer basis, carry out their nursing within their own faith communities. This is usually desirable for both nurse and congregation, because the parish nurse is thus familiar with the spiritual and religious beliefs of the congregation and of the pastor. In the future, however, if parish nursing becomes "professionalized" to a greater degree, and if acceptable to a faith community, parish nurses may be hired to work with a church not of their own denomination. This kind of partnering does exist to some degree, in contemporary hospital-based parish nursing programs in which staff parish nurses provide consultation and support to developing church programs from a variety of religious traditions.

In this era of continued change within the U.S. health care system, including such factors as short hospital stays, same day surgeries, and early discharges, parish nursing, or nursing provided to those in their homes by members of a local faith community, may be critical to a patient's recovery, and perhaps even to his or her survival. No longer are patients, especially older patients or those who live alone, allowed the luxury of remaining in the hospital until they are able to fully function on their own. Health insurance policies rarely cover such extended stays, even if a patient's recovery may be at risk. It is expected that many of the former hospital nursing care services will now be provided by relatives or friends in a home care setting. This makes the role of the contemporary parish nurse vitally important to recovering patients who have no extended family networks and who may depend on their churches for caring support in times of crisis or significant need. It is suggested that individuals of all ages can benefit from the "personal caring and attention offered by a parish nursing model" (Stewart, 2000, p. 116).

One of the first things a parish nurse may find helpful in beginning to work with a faith community, especially a church to which the concept of parish nursing is new, is to do a "needs assessment" of the parish. There are a variety of needs assessment schemas being developed; however, the assessment must take into account certain factors that vary in parishes, such as the mean age of the parishioners, the range of socioeconomic levels in the church, the parish size, and the availability of volunteers to assist with the development of a parish health ministry. Parish nurses report that a critical factor in beginning a new effort with a faith community is the support of the pastor; as noted above, he or she may have concerns about the time, financial, and/or legal burdens that the establishment of any new program may bring to the church. If however, the potential parish nurse or health ministry team can predict that the program will be a benefit rather than a burden to the church, most pastors are enthusiastic in their support of the effort.

Although existing church-based parish nursing programs are still new to many faith communities, the number and scope of these ministries is expanding rapidly. In some churches, programs may be limited to such activities as monthly blood-pressure screenings, with occasional health educational programs for the congregation and infrequent home or hospital visiting by members of an "on-call" volunteer team; there may or may not be a parish nurse leading the effort. In other parishes, well-developed parish health ministry programs exist, under the leadership of a paid part-time or full-time parish or congregational nurse.

Depending on the interest and sophistication, in terms of health care experience, on the part of a pastor and congregation, a church may require that their parish nurse have specific training in parish nursing; be a nurse practitioner; have a number of years of experience in nursing; or simply be a registered nurse who has a commitment and desire to work with a faith community. For example, one church in a moderately sized urban area advertised for a part-time parish nurse who would be a licensed RN in the state with at least three years experience in nursing; the church also wanted the candidate to have completed a parish nursing preparation course, although the parameters of that course were not specified. It was noted that the nurse's role would include health promotion, disease prevention, education, counseling, advocacy, health screening, and referral. The parish nurse's hours could be "flexible."

Some congregations employing either paid or volunteer parish nurses try to schedule "office hours" at the parish, for example, Wednesdays and Fridays, 9–12 noon, so that parishioners can come for private consultation or education. In such a situation the parish nurse will usually have "on call" hours also. Some of the activities associated with existing parish nursing or health ministry programs, in addition to parish nurse office hours and monthly BP screening, include exercise classes (especially for seniors), CPR classes, foot care classes, nutritional education classes, diabetes education classes, prenatal classes, bike safety classes for children, self breast exam classes, substance abuse classes for parents and teens, healthy aging classes, family fitness classes, and classes preparing church volunteers for such ministries as hospital and nursing home visiting, homebound visiting, and respite family care.

The parish nurse may him/herself also do some home and hospital visiting as time permits; the nurse's most important role, however, is to serve as the health ministry team leader and coordinator of non-medical health ministry volunteers. The parish nurse is an advocate for the ill parishioners of a faith community and a source of referral to needed and appropriate community health services.

(Note: Following are a "Parish Health Needs Assessment" form and six tables of guidelines which may be useful for parish nurses initiating health ministry programs.)

Parish Health Needs Assessment

> *Come, you that are blessed by my Father, inherit the king-dom prepared for you from the foundation of the world . . . for I was . . . sick and you took care of me.*

MATTHEW 25:34–35

Introduction: The purpose of this parish health needs assessment questionnaire is to help [church name]'s parish nursing/health ministry team identify priorities in planning activities for the ministry. All information will be kept confidential; placing your name and address on the questionnaire is purely OPTIONAL.

A. *Personal Data (Optional)*
 1. Name _____
    Address _____
    Phone # _____ E-mail _____
B. *Demographic Data and Personal Health History*
 2. Age _____ 3. Gender _____
 4. Marital Status   Single ○ Married ○
    Widowed ○ Divorced ○ Separated ○
 5. Household Members (who you live with)
    Alone _____
    Spouse _____
    Spouse and Children _____
    Adult Children _____
    Minor Children _____
    Other Relatives/Friends _____
 6. Frequency of Church Attendance
    Daily ○   More than once a week ○
    Once a week ○   Once a month ○
    Less than once a month ○ 2 to 3 times a year ○
    Never ○
 7. Occupation (current/former) _____

8. Employment Status
   Full-time ○   Part-time ○   Retired ○
   Volunteer ○ (Specify number of hours per week) _____
9. Primary Illness Diagnosis (if any) _____
10. Disability (if any)
11. Current Medications or Treatments (if any)
12. Other Diagnoses (please specify if any)
    Respiratory Conditions (e.g., COPD)
    Neurological Conditions (e.g., stroke)
    Psychiatric Conditions (e.g., depression)
    Circulatory Conditions (e.g., heart disease)
    Musculoskeletal Conditions (e.g., arthritis)
    Endocrine Conditions (e.g., diabetes)
    Gastrointestinal Conditions (e.g., reflux)
    Integumentary (skin) Conditions (e.g., dermatitis)
    Other Diagnosis(es)
13. Please specify any other medical or illness history that you would like the church health ministry team to know about:

    _____

    _____

C. *Specific Health/Illness-Related Needs*
   1. Physical needs in the home (e.g., shopping; preparing meals)

      _____

   2. Psychosocial needs at home (e.g., companionship; assistance with letter writing)

      _____

      _____

   3. Spiritual needs at home (e.g., visit from a spiritual minister; prayer; the sacraments)

      _____

      _____

   4. Health education/counseling at home (e.g., diabetic teaching)

      _____

      _____

5. Legal advice at home (e.g., preparing a will; advance directives)

_____

6. Transportation (e.g., to physician's office; church; grocery store)

_____

7. Family respite assistance

_____

D. *Suggested health promotion workshops that you would like to see the church's health ministry sponsor:*
   1. Women's Health Issues
   2. Men's Health Issues
   3. Teen Addictions/Eating Disorders
   4. Aging with Grace
   5. Healthy Nutrition and Exercise
   6. Stress Reduction Techniques
   7. Diabetes Education
   8. Alzheimer's Disease
   9. Medicare and Medicaid Insurance
   10. Advance Directives (Living Wills)
   11. Coping with Grief and Bereavement
   12. The Relationship between Faith and Health

E. *Suggestions for/response to the church's support of the parish nursing/health ministry initiative:*

_____

_____

Thank you for completing this questionnaire. Please feel free to add additional comments in the space below as desired.

God bless you,
 The Parish Nursing/Health Ministry Team
of [church name]'s Church

Table 10.1 Guidelines for Developing a Parish Health Ministry Program

1. Describe the role of the parish health minister.
2. Explain the biblical spirituality of the parish health minister's vocation.
3. State who may become a parish health minister.
4. Specify the kind of training/orientation required to become a parish health minister.
5. Give examples of potential parish health ministry activities.
6. Share a statement of support for the ministry from the church pastor (and other clergy or church leaders, if appropriate).
7. Broadly describe who the potential recipients of parish health ministry might be.
8. Identify a parish contact person (usually a parish nurse) with whom parishioners interested in parish health ministry might consult.
9. Present a brief description of the commissioning ceremony for parish health ministers (if appropriate) as a formal validation of a parishioner's response to God's call to serve.

Table 10.2 Suggested Activities for Parish Health Ministers

1. Home, hospital, and nursing home/assisted care facility visitation

   Praying with parishioners

   Bringing holy Communion (if appropriate)

   Reading scripture or other spiritual books

   Listening and visiting with parishioners; sharing news of the church or other areas of interest

   Counseling/advising on spiritual/health-related issues (as appropriate)

2. Running errands such as grocery shopping or picking up prescriptions (for homebound elders)

3. Phone ministry to homebound parishioners

4. Providing periods of respite for family caregivers

5. Writing notes/holiday cards to parishioners who are hospitalized, homebound, or living in nursing homes/ assisted care facilities

6. Writing parish health ministry articles for the church bulletin

7. Assisting with the planning and coordinating of health education programs for the congregation

8. Assisting with organizing and coordinating health promotion programs such as blood pressure screening

9. Organizing a prayer partner program for the church

10. Organizing and maintaining a loan closet of healthcare supplies for ill or disabled parishioners

11. Planning and coordinating a church health fair

12. Communicating with other interested parishioners about the health ministry and its needs

Table 10.3 Parish Health Ministry Visits to Homebound Parishioners

1. Check with the parishioner or family about a convenient time to visit.
2. Prior to the visit, ask whether the ill parishioner has any visual, hearing, or speech impairments.
3. Seek to determine areas of the parishioner's interest for a pastoral visit, such as Holy Communion, prayer, scripture reading, spiritual counseling, or health counseling.
4. Listen actively; allow the parishioner to talk about things that are important to him or her.
5. Bring Holy Communion (if appropriate), a Bible, and a list of local community healthcare resources (if appropriate).
6. Draw the visit to a conclusion if parishioner begins to appear fatigued.
7. Begin and end the health ministry visit with prayer.

Table 10.4 Parish Health Ministry Visits to Hospitalized Parishioners

1. Call the parishioner or family to find out whether a parish health ministry visit is desired or acceptable.
2. Check with hospital staff to identify appropriate visiting hours (and visitor restrictions/time limitations), especially for areas such as intensive care.
3. Be aware of possible ministry visit interruptions related to medical/nursing interventions.
4. Be alert to parishioner–patient's level of energy/fatigue (don't overstay a visit).
5. Pray with the patient (and family, if present) at the beginning and the end of the visit.

Table 10.5 Parish Health Ministry to Parishioners Residing in Long-Term Care Facilities

1. Check with the resident or facility staff for appropriate visiting times.
2. Arrive when expected by the resident (elders, especially, look forward to visitors with much anticipation).
3. Plan to spend enough time, during which the resident can share problems and concerns, if needed; loneliness is a prevailing issue in long-term care facilities.
4. Visit facility-bound residents on major holidays if possible (these are particularly lonely times for elders with little or no family to take them home for a visit).
5. Begin and end the visit with prayer.

Table 10.6 Parish Health Ministry Visits to Terminally Ill Parishioners and Bereaved Family Members

1. Listen! Listen! Listen! Dying persons and bereaved family members very much need to talk to someone who cares.
2. Don't preach! Allow the Holy Spirit to do that through the ministry and caring of your visit.
3. Be gentle in response to anger (if manifested). As a representative of the Church, and of God, you might be faced with hostility related to a parishioner's pain.
4. Be present! Don't give up unless you are asked to leave. A dying person and a bereaved individual are both experiencing loss; they may need to work through frustrations and anger in the presence of a caring minister.
5. Pray at the beginning and end of the visit.

Parish nursing is presently a developing subfield within the larger nursing community, but interest in the area is growing rapidly. New parish nursing education programs continue to be developed by colleges and universities and by church-related organizations. It is hoped that eventually there will be ANA certification for parish nurses. Until this comes about, however, professional nurses who feel called by God to serve within a faith community continue to support and enhance the parish nursing role through their vision and their dedication. The concept of parish nursing is very new and it is also very old; contemporary parish nurses have embraced their ministry with the caring and commitment of the first century deacons and deaconesses, and with the wisdom and understanding of present-day nursing knowledge. Parish nursing, however it develops in the coming decades, is definitely here to stay.

A Nurse's Prayer for Wisdom

Dear Father,
It's so easy to forget, in the
busyness of the day, all that your
Son has taught; thank you for
sending the Spirit, in His Name,
　　　　　　(John 14:26)
to "remind" us of the beauty and the power of Jesus'
gospel message of caring and compassion.

For it is only through the teaching of the Spirit:
that our parish nurses' hearts will be moved to love;
that our parish nurses' minds will be inspired to counsel;
that our parish nurses' thoughts will be directed to educate;
that our parish nurses' souls will be guided to pray.

Bless us, Lord God of our lives,
with the teaching that will bring us to true understanding
through the grace of Him, who alone, is the
Spirit of Truth and wisdom.

References

Dunkle, R. E. (2000). Parish nurses help patients, body and soul. In R. Hunt (Ed.), *Readings in Community Based Nursing* (pp. 316–320). Philadelphia: Lippincott.

(2001). FAQ about HMA & parish nursing. *Connections, The Health Ministries Association Information & Contacts*, 1(2), 1.

Lovinus, B. (1996). A healer in the midst of the congregation. *The Journal of Christian Healing*, 18(4), 3–18.

McDermott, M., Solari-Twadell, P., & Matheus, R. (1999). Educational preparation. In P. Solari-Twadell and M. McDermott (Eds.), *Parish Nursing: Promoting Whole Person Health within Faith Communities* (pp. 269–276). Thousand Oaks, CA: Sage Publications.

Palmer, J. (2001). Parish nursing: Connecting faith and health. *Reflections on Nursing Leadership*, 27(1), 17–19; 45–46.

(1998). *Scope and standards of parish nursing practice*. Washington, D.C.: American Nurses Publishing.

Solari-Twadell, P., & Westberg, G. (1991). Body, mind and soul: The parish nurse offers physical, emotional and spiritual care. *Health Progress*, 72(7), 24–28.

Stewart, L. E. (2000). Parish nursing: Reviewing a long tradition of caring. *Gastroenterology Nursing*, 23(3), 16–20.

Westberg, G. (1990). *The parish nurse: Providing a minister of health for your congregation*. Minneapolis, MN: Augsburg.

Zerson, D. (1994). Parish nursing: 20th century fad? *Journal of Christian Nursing*, 11(2), 19–22.

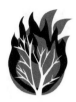

CHAPTER II

Spiritual Care in Mass Casualty Disasters

I have called you by name, you are mine. When you pass through the waters, I will be with you; and through the rivers, they shall not overwhelm you; when you walk through fire you shall not be burned, and the flames shall not consume you.

ISAIAH 43:1-2

The Prayer of a Wounded Healer

The wounds are many, Dear Lord, and deep.
I bruise so easily; it's always been that way.
Most of the scars have healed, or so it seems.
They're barely visible to the eye now; but
to the heart, well, that's another matter.

Sometimes, when I least suspect, an ache begins
somewhere far down.
It grows into a hurt that burns my throat,
as I try valiantly to master the tears begging to be shed.

I grab for the nearest Band-Aid,
seeking desperately to stem the bleeding;
but nothing heals except Your love,

Dear Lord.
I'm so tired of trying to pretend it's otherwise.

And, so, I come humbly to You,
in prayer; a healer wounded
in heart and in spirit.
You anoint my scars with the Blessed tears of
Your Son and they are transformed
and made beautiful.

Teach me, Dear Lord, to appreciate
these liberating wounds, which open my nurse's
heart to the pain of my sorrowful and suffering patients.

Teach me, Dear Lord, to accept these
hidden wounds, which help me to understand
the loneliness of my poor and marginalized patients.

Teach me, Dear Lord, to cherish these
tender wounds, which fill me with compassion for the
anxiety of my frightened and hopeless patients.

Teach me, Beloved Wounded Healer, to
learn of You, that I may become
myself a healer, wounded
yet healed, to be for the injured
an instrument of Your healing
and Your love.

This chapter begins with a brief overview of disaster nursing, including the types and phases of disasters, and selected key disaster service agencies: the Federal Emergency Management Agency (FEMA), the American Red Cross, and the Salvation Army. Following are discussions of the psychosocial impact of mass casualty trauma, spiritual needs in the aftermath of a disaster, and the nurse's role in the spiritual care of disaster victims.

Disaster Nursing

Most books on the topic of disaster nursing were published in the era of the mid-twentieth century, the 1950s and 1960s. They included concerns about disasters such as hurricanes, tornados, fires, floods, accidents, and nuclear radiation incidents, such as those caused by an atomic bomb explosion. Although there was some discussion of biological and chemical warfare, the concept of suicidal terrorist attacks, as occurred in the United States on September 11, 2001, were not considered. Although these earlier disaster nursing books do include discussions of the psychosocial impact of a disaster, spiritual or religious needs in mass casualty trauma are not included as key topics of discussion. In that era, the assessment of a patient or family member's spiritual or religious need was still considered by many nurses to fall within the role of the pastoral caregiver only; that thinking has changed, and a number of nurses have developed spiritual assessment scales to be used as nursing tools.

Disaster nursing poses multiple challenges in terms of assessment and intervention. Most disaster scenes also include elements of danger and confusion; thus, the "physical and emotional stress factors may be extreme" (Brown, 1985, p. 45). Although disaster nursing is a unique area of nursing, only a modest number of journal articles on the topic are found in the literature; this is probably related to the fact that the majority of nurses have never had disaster nursing experience and never expect to become engaged in such nursing. A disaster has been described as "any man-made or natural event that causes destruction and devastation and that cannot be alleviated without assistance" (Hassmiller, 2000, p. 401), and as testing "the adaptive responses of communities or individuals beyond their capabilities and lead[ing] to at least a temporary disruption of function" (Clark, 1999, p. 704). Disasters are generally categorized as falling within two broad categories: natural disasters, such as tornadoes, hurricanes, floods, avalanches, earthquakes, volcanic eruptions, and communicable diseases; and human-generated disasters, including warfare, riots, mass demonstrations, and accidents (Lundy & Butts, 2001, p. 551). A disaster is classified as a "multiple patient incident" if less than ten casualties have occurred; as a "multiple casualty incident" if there are less than 100 casualties but stress is placed on local health care facilities; and as a "mass casualty incident or disaster" if the occurrence involves over 100 casualties and "significantly overtaxes existing health care facilities" (Demi & Miles, 1984, p. 64).

Disaster phases have been identified in various ways, including such stages as predisaster preparation, warning, impact, emergency, and recovery (Taggart, 1985, p. 7); and prevention, preparedness, response, and recovery (Tait and Spradley, 2001, p. 394). Regardless of terminology, the disaster phases are generally considered to include some period of disaster planning or preparation, a time of immediate impact and emergency response, and a recovery period. It is important to remember that nurses involved in responding to a disaster impact may themselves be victims of the disaster, especially if the incident involves an entire community, as in the case of a tornado or flood. Often the nurse will have to put personal or family concerns on a "back burner," to carry out his or her professional responsibilities.

The nurse's role in a disaster response may depend on where the nurse happens to be at the time of impact, such as at home, a hospital, a clinic, or somewhere in the community. If a nurse is in the immediate location of the disaster, he or she may be able to make a direct nursing response through such activities as "assisting in evacuation, rescue, and first aid efforts until the immediate needs of the situation are met" (Taggert, 1985, p. 11).

As noted, there may be a multiplicity of first aid and other emergency care needs at a disaster site that will fall within the purview of the nurse. Some related activities that professional nurses might assist with include providing leadership; maintaining a communication network; organizing the provision of food, warmth, shelter, and social support; and counseling victims who appear to display "panic or hysterical behavior" (Reichsmeier & Miller, 1985, p. 191). Another important role of the nurse responding to a disaster situation is awareness and assessment of the needs of the rescue workers. If the disaster is particularly devastating in terms of multiple injuries or loss of life, "psychological reactions can easily overwhelm relief teams of caregivers unless careful attention is given to meeting basic biological needs, especially the need for rest and sleep" (Reichsmeier & Miller, 1985, p. 199).

Disaster Services

Three agencies are charged with the provision of relief services in mass casualty disasters in the United States: the Federal Emergency Management Agency (FEMA), the American Red Cross, and the Salvation Army. Each group has specific responsibilities in times of disaster and mass trauma.

Federal Emergency Management Agency (FEMA)

The Federal Emergency Management Agency (FEMA) is an independent agency of the federal government that is charged with planning for and responding to disasters, both natural and man made. The organization "has also been active in the development of nationwide contingency systems for disaster relief" (Switzer, 1985, p. 318). FEMA staff provide leadership in recovery efforts and support to the victims of disasters through both direct and indirect funding of services to provide the necessities of daily life and functioning. FEMA, founded in 1979, has a staff of several thousand full-time workers, supported by reservists who can be activated if needed. FEMA is called in whenever a situation is declared a disaster or in need of emergency services.

The American Red Cross

The American Red Cross, initiated under the direction of nurse Clara Barton in 1881, received its charge from the 58th Congress of the United States to "continue and carry on a system of national and international relief in time of . . . suffering caused by pestilence, famine, fire, floods and other great national calamities" (Nabbe, 1961, p. 10). Thus, the American Red Cross, although not a government agency, has a national mandate to provide relief services in times of great calamity and disaster in our country; the group is also mandated to provide services for the armed forces of the country as needed. The Red Cross is primarily a volunteer organization supported by private contributions and the volunteer work of a number of individuals. A significant role of the American Red Cross is the provision of blood supplies to hospitals in need of supplemental stocks for disaster victims. Other activities carried out by Red Cross nursing staff and volunteers include providing first aid at disaster sites, feeding rescue and recovery workers, providing food and shelter for disaster victims, communicating with families of disaster victims, providing mental health services, and assisting survivors with accessing available resources. The Red Cross suggests that "community health skills and psychological support skills are important assets for a nurse to possess when helping victims after a disaster" (Hanson, Jesz, & Baldwin, 1991, p. 391).

The Salvation Army

The Salvation Army is an international religious organization founded in London in 1865 by William Booth. The "Army" adopted, early on, a military style of organization and dress; this reflects the group's war against evil as well as its witness of the Christian gospel, to which all army members adhere. Many people think of Salvation Army members primarily as the "bell-ringers," seen on city street corners with their classic red collection buckets. In fact, this activity of collecting money for the poor is only a small part of the Army's ministry. As well as carrying out a number of services for those in need, the Salvation Army embraces the commitment of assisting any community following a disaster incident. Army members can usually be seen at disaster sites involved in such works as feeding survivors and rescue workers, counseling those in need of psychological and social support, providing grief and bereavement counseling, praying with persons desiring spiritual support, and generally assisting victims and their families with whatever needs they present, in attempting to cope with the disaster experience and its aftermath.

Psychosocial Impact of Mass Casualty Trauma

Support provided by the above identified organizations is critical in managing a mass casualty trauma, because in such situations, the problems, especially the psychosocial problems experienced by both victims and responders, frequently "exceed the medical community's resources to deal with them" (Baker, 1980, p. 149). Two broad categories of disaster victims are identified: primary victims, who "directly experience physical, material and personal losses from the disaster event"; and secondary victims, who "witness the destructiveness of the disaster but do not experience the actual impact" (Bolin, 1985, p. 6). Secondary victims may include both family members and rescue workers involved in a disaster incident. The American Psychiatric Association's DSM IV Classification now identifies "bearing witness to a trauma or being confronted by the traumatic experience of a family member or close friend" as a stressor that may have "psychiatric consequences"

(Fullerton & Ursano, 1997, p. 59). It has been found that a disaster may impact not only a victim's sense of physical security, but also faith in the goodness of God and humankind. Thus, a disaster has important implications for spiritual need and spiritual care.

Spiritual Needs in the Aftermath of a Disaster

The topic of spiritual needs immediately after, and in the long term following, a mass casualty disaster is vast. A disaster victim's or a responder's spiritual needs may involve a desire for personal prayer or prayer with a clergy person; a loving hug or words of support from a relative, friend, or caregiver; formal religious rituals in cases of death or critical wounding of loved ones; and myriad other kinds of spiritual or religious support. Much will have to do with the nature of the disaster, the role of the individual in the disaster, and the personal spiritual or religious orientation of the victim or responder. Examples of need and kind of spiritual/religious care provided are best presented in context of a specific disaster incident.

The Disaster Nurse's Role in Spiritual Care

Perhaps the most important thing that a nurse caring for a disaster victim can do, in terms of spiritual care, is to reinforce the fact that the trauma a patient has experienced was not caused by God, or brought about by any behavior on the victim's part. This can free a victim from possible feelings of guilt, help restore his or her faith in God, and allow the individual to turn to God for help in overcoming the suffering caused by the disaster. Before attempting to provide more specific spiritual care such as praying with a patient or clergy referral, a nurse can do an on-the-spot spiritual assessment by asking a few simple questions related to a disaster victim's spiritual or religious tradition, such as finding out what kind of pastoral care or prayer life they have been used to and what might support them both immediately and in future coping with the disaster. Family members, if available, can provide much of this information. Also, a variety of volunteer clergy members are usually present at disaster sites; their intervention may be very helpful in assisting the nurse with both assessment and planning for a patient's future, especially if the victim is to be hospitalized.

As suggested in Chapter 2, not all nurses will or need to feel comfortable in providing such spiritual care as praying with a patient; they may, however, feel at ease giving a supportive hug. Nurses in disaster situations should, however, be prepared to assess a patient's spiritual needs, especially if the victim is seriously or mortally wounded. For example, a critically injured Roman Catholic victim would be greatly comforted to receive an anointing or "the Sacrament of the Sick"; this could be done on the spot, if a priest is available. It is doubtful that any priest would come to a disaster site without bringing the holy oil needed for the sacrament. If the patient should die either at the disaster site or in transport to a hospital, the fact that the "last rites" of the Church had been administered prior to his or her death would be very meaningful to a Catholic family.

It can also be helpful for a disaster nurse to provide clergy referral to less seriously injured victims for future spiritual care and counseling. It is very important to refer patients to pastors who are willing and able to listen to the sometimes graphic and gruesome reports of a disaster scene "in a nonjudgmental and practical way but with a sensitivity to the theological implications for the victim" (Williams, 1998, p. 330). Because of the "trust many people have in ministers" they often become natural crisis counselors (Clinebell, 1991, p. 183). Nurses also are "natural crisis counselors" and natural providers of spiritual care, because they are often the people most closely involved with a victim immediately after a disaster. Guidelines suggested for pastoral caregivers working with trauma victims can also be useful for disaster nurses regarding the provision of spiritual support and spiritual care; some of these include "non-judgmental acceptance of

the survivor," a posture of "support and advocacy," an understanding of "posttraumatic distress," "willingness to be exposed to
the survivor's recounting of the traumatic experience," and recognition that grieving may be a lifelong process (Foy, Drescher, Fitz,
& Kennedy, 1993, p. 631). The authors also note that the spiritual caregiver should provide for "pastoral self-care" (p. 631).
Pastoral or spiritual self-care is a given for any nurse attempting to
provide spiritual care for victims of a mass casualty disaster.

The topic of spiritual need in mass casualty disasters is vast and
variable. Spiritual needs in the immediate and long-term periods
following a disaster are very much related to the particular disaster incident and to the overall needs of the victims and their families. Little had been written on the spirituality of disaster nursing
prior to September 11, 2001; I found virtually nothing in the early
nursing literature specifically exploring the spiritual needs of the
survivors. Following the terrible pain and suffering of 9/11, nurses have begun to explore the topics of spiritual need and spiritual
care in mass casualty trauma. These topics, related, specifically to
the 9/11 "Attack on America," are discussed in my book,
Spirituality in Nursing: Standing on Holy Ground (O'Brien, 2003).

A Nurse's Prayer to Become a Healer

> *All in the crowd were trying to touch him, for power came*
> *forth from him and HEALED all of them.*

> LUKE 6:19

> O God, who heals our hurts and calms our fears with the
> passion of Your love, teach me to be a healer. Gift my
> nursing that it may be blessed with the soothing balm of
> a tender touch, the comforting peace of a caring spirit,
> and the healing grace of a loving heart. Help me to step
> out with the courage and compassion of the healer
> Veronica, as I tenderly minister to the ill and the infirm.

May I never forget to see, in the countenance of each person I serve, the Blessed image of Your Divine Son. Amen.

References

Baker, F. J. (1980). The management of mass casualty disasters. In H. W. Meislin (Ed.), *Priorities in multiple trauma* (pp. 149–157). Germantown, MD: Aspen Systems.

Bolin, R. (1985). Disaster characteristics and psychosocial impacts. In B. J. Sowder (Ed.), *Disasters and mental health: Selected contemporary perspectives* (pp. 3–28). Rockville, MD: National Institutes of Mental Health.

Brown, R. L. (1985). Management and triage at the disaster site. In L. M. Garcia (Ed.), *Disaster nursing: Planning, assessment and intervention* (pp. 45–70). Rockville, MD: Aspen Systems.

Clark, M. J. (1999). *Nursing in the community*. Stamford, CT: Appleton & Lange.

Clinebell, H. (1991). *Basic types of pastoral care and counseling*. Nashville, TN: Abingdon Press.

Demi, A., & Miles, M. S. (1984). An examination of nursing leadership following a disaster. *Topics in Clinical Nursing, 6*(1), 63–78.

Foy, D. A., Drescher, K. D., Fitz, A. G., & Kennedy, K. R. (1993). Posttraumatic stress disorder. In R. J. Wicks and R. D. Parsons (Eds.), *Clinical handbook of pastoral counseling, volume 2* (pp. 621–637). Mahwah, NJ: Paulist Press.

Fullerton, C. S., & Ursano, R. J. (1997). Posttraumatic responses in spouse/significant others of disaster workers. In C. S. Fullerton & R. J. Ursano (Eds.), *Posttraumatic stress disorder: Acute and long term responses to trauma and disaster* (pp. 59–75). Washington, DC: American Psychiatric Press.

Hanson, C., Jesz, B. L., & Baldwin, S. S. (1991). The American Red Cross: A nursing oriented overview of services. *Journal of Emergency Nursing, 17*(6), 390, 394.

Hassmiller, S. B. (2000). Disaster management. In M. Stanhope and J. Lancaster (Eds.), *Community and public health nursing* (pp. 400–415). St. Louis: Mosby.

Lundy, K. S., & Butts, J. B. (2001). The role of the community health nurse in disasters. In K. S. Lundy and S. Janes (Eds.). *Community health nursing: Caring for the public's health* (pp. 546–573). Sudbury, MA: Jones and Bartlett Publishers.

Nabbe, F. C. (1961). *Disaster nursing*. Paterson, NJ: Littlefield, Adams & Company.

O'Brien, M.E. (2003) *Spirituality in nursing: Standing on holy ground.* Sudbury, MA: Jones and Bartlett Publishers.

Reichsmeier, J. L., & Miller, J. K. (1985). Psychological aspects of disaster situations. In L. M. Garcia (Ed.), *Disaster nursing: Planning, assessment and intervention* (pp. 185–202). Rockville, MD: Aspen Systems.

Switzer, K. H. (1985). Disaster planning: Assessing and using community resources. In L. M. Garcia (Ed.), *Disaster nursing: Planning, assessment and intervention* (pp. 307–344). Rockville, MD: Aspen Systems.

Taggert, S. B. (1985). Background and historical perspective. In L. M. Garcia (Ed.), *Disaster nursing: Planning, assessment and intervention* (pp. 1–16). Rockville, MD: Aspen Systems.

Tait, C., & Spradley, B. (2001). Communities in crisis: Disasters, group violence and terrorism. In J. A. Allender & B. W. Spradley (Eds.), *Community health nursing: Concepts and practice* (pp. 391–407). Philadelphia: Lippincott.

Williams, T. (1998). Diagnosis and treatment of survivor guilt. In J. P. Wilson, Z. Harel, & B. Kahana (Eds.), *Human adaptation to extreme stress* (pp. 319–336). New York: Plenum Press.

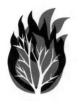

CHAPTER 12

Prayer in Nursing: The Spirituality of Compassionate Caregiving

When you call upon me, and come and pray to me, I will listen to you.

JEREMIAH 29:12

The Nurse: God's Vessel

Vessels hold all kinds of blessed things:
food and drink to nourish the body;
candles and perfumes to nourish the spirit;
the light of Christ to nourish the soul.

Vessels are treasured when empty; they can be filled.
Vessels are precious when full; they can be emptied.
Vessels may break; they can be mended,
stronger, often, for the sealing of the breach.

Nurses are called to be God's vessels:
to be empty, awaiting the fullness of His love;
to be full, awaiting the emptiness of self-giving;
to be broken, in the service of the sick;
to be stronger, for the healing of the wound.

In a small but powerful book on prayer, Benedictine Mary Clare Vincent observed "a life without prayer doesn't work." (Vincent, 1982, p. 1) I would add that nursing without prayer doesn't work. For contemporary nurses, prayer is, I believe, more necessary to support their caring for the sick than in any preceding era. Complex moral and ethical issues, related both directly and tangentially to our practice, abound in the current world of health care. Therapeutic procedures involving a variety of extraordinary measures to prolong human life (some of which are admittedly positive) become more sophisticated each year; and medical research on such frightening issues as cloning of human beings hovers on the fringe of acceptable medical discourse in certain quarters.

If, in fact, we subscribe to the spiritual vision of our profession's founder, how can we not believe in the importance and value of prayer for a nurse? For it was Florence Nightingale who reminded us, in the late nineteenth century, that "God's precious gift of life is often placed literally in [the nurse's] hands." (Nightingale, 1859, pp. 70–71) What a sacred commission Nightingale issued to her followers—to hold in our hands "God's precious gift of life." How can we be faithful to such a blessed ministry without the grace of prayer? And yet, in this era of health care reform, of managed care and restructured nursing roles, what does prayer mean for the contemporary nurse? How can time for prayer be found in a caregiving system in which all activities must be cost effective, as mandated by the institutions in which we carry out our nursing activities? The purpose of this book is to address these and related questions and concerns for present day nurses; the ultimate goal is to explore the practice of prayerful, compassionate caregiving in the world of twenty-first-century nursing.

Reclaiming Our Spiritual Heritage: A History of Prayer in Nursing

From its inception, nursing the sick has been considered a vocation or calling; in the early days, especially, nursing was viewed as a ministry of God and of His Church and was guided and strengthened by the prayer of the caregiver. Our nursing forebears, on whose strong shoulders we contemporary nurses stand, understood this calling; they responded by including prayer as a central and critical component of their nursing ministries. In the book *Spirituality in Nursing: Standing on Holy Ground*, I devoted an entire chapter to the spiritual history of nursing. Tales of nursing prefigures from the early deacons and deaconesses of the first century, through the medieval monastics such as Hildegard of Bingen and St. Francis of Assisi, up to members of the post-reformation religious orders, are replete with anecdotes indicating the prayerfulness with which nursing ministries were undertaken (O'Brien, 2003, pp. 21–54). For these men and women, committed to a religious vocation of caring for the sick, God's call, heard in prayer, not only was the incentive for undertaking the ministry but also was the very fiber from which a daily tapestry of nursing activities was woven.

In the mid-nineteenth century, Florence Nightingale's life and writings modeled a variety of prayers. In a letter to her Aunt Hannah, written in 1846, Florence described her prayer of petition: "I never pray for anything temporal . . . but when each morning comes, I kneel down before the Rising Sun and only say: 'Behold the handmaid of the Lord, give me this day my work to do, no, not my work, but Thine.'" (Dossey, 2000, p. 33) A Nightingale diary entry acknowledges the author's listening to the Lord in prayer: "God called me in the morning and asked me: 'Would I do good for Him, for Him alone without reputation [self-interest].'" (Dossey, p. 65) Florence's mystical bent and her gift for contemplation are reflected in a famous quote from *Notes for Devotional Authors*: "Where shall I find God? In myself. That is the true mystical doctrine. But then I myself must be in a state for Him to come and dwell in me." (Macrae, 1995, p. 10)

In a qualitative study of spirituality and nursing, which I conducted among 66 contemporary nurses, the importance of prayer in the nurse's practice was demonstrated graphically in a theme labeled "Nursing Liturgy." A touching example is an anecdote shared by a pediatric nurse practitioner who described a prayerful "nursing liturgy" carried out prior to the death of an anencephalic newborn:

> The baby, a "preemie," had lived for a couple of weeks, but there were so many congenital anomalies that there was no hope; so the family signed the papers to terminate life support. The parents just couldn't be there, though, so we decided to plan something. It was a very young neonatologist; it was really hard on him, and myself and the Peds ICU head nurse. We came into the NICU (Neonatal Intensive Care Unit) at about 5 A.M. on a Saturday, when there weren't a lot of staff around. We took the baby into a separate little isolation room and discontinued the "vent" and the IVs, all the life support systems. And then we prayed and we sang hymns and we just held her and loved her until she died. It was her special ritual to go to God, and we shared it with her. (O'Brien, 2003, pp. 107–108)

The Use of Scripture for Prayer in Nursing

There is a multiplicity of spiritual books to assist in the exercise of praying with Scripture such as *Pray the Bible* by Page Zyromski; (Zyromski, 2000) and many relevant chapters in books on prayer, for example "Listening at Prayer with the Written Word"; (Groeschel, 1984) "Pondering the Word"; (Casey, 1996) and "Contemplating Scripture." (Barry, 1987) There are also bible dictionaries and commentaries that help explain the meaning of more obscure scripture passages, as well as providing the history of the holy word; one simple and useful example is the *Collegeville Series on Books of the Bible*. (Liturgical Press, 1987).

For many of us, it may be easier to begin with the New Testament—with Scriptures familiar from our worship services: the four gospels; the Acts of the Apostles; and the letters of Jesus' disciples: Paul, James, Peter, John, and Jude. Or we may wish to pick an Old Testament passage with which we also have some familiarity such as the story of Jeremiah and the Potter's Wheel (Jeremiah 18: 1–6), or the prophet Isaiah's promise that those who hope in the Lord will "soar as with eagle's wings" (Isaiah 40: 31). The Psalms are also a wonderful guide to prayer as they are the prayers that Jesus prayed. Each psalm has a unique theme that might be relevant to a particular prayer concern such as praise, thanksgiving, trust; prayer in time of illness; prayer in distress; confidence in God; prayer for help against unjust enemies; prayer for protection; and prayer for faithfulness. Finally, to identify those scripture passages that may be helpful in prayer, a concordance or dictionary of scripture references is a wonderful guide to finding one's way around the books of the Bible.

Finding Time for Prayer in Nursing: An "Oratory of the Heart"

Brother Lawrence of the Resurrection, sometimes called "saint of the pots and pans," asserted: "It is not necessary for being with God to be always at church. We may make an oratory of our heart wherein to retire from time to time to converse with him." (Brother Lawrence, 1973, p. 48) Other scholars of prayer suggest that we may incorporate prayer into our busy days by such activities as thinking of God as we are walking about or working at some manual task; praying the "Jesus Prayer," using a brief formula such as "Come Lord Jesus" or simply repeating the name of Jesus; and meditating on the holiness of ordinary tasks, especially those involving the care of a brother or sister in need. Nursing practice, in its many and varied dimensions, surely lends itself to the latter kind of prayerful meditation.

A strategy that helps me to try to pray even when I am too busy, is to decorate my living and work spaces with spiritual/religious pictures and thoughts. I also have a beautifully carved wooden crucifix on my office wall, given to me many years ago when I entered religious life; and a print of Domenico Fetti's 1622 oil painting entitled *The Veil of Veronica*, which one of my students brought me from the National Gallery of Art. Above my computer is a special favorite, a framed print of Jean-Francois Millet's magnificently prayerful painting *The Angelus*. The mid-nineteenth-century scene depicts two young farmers, standing heads bent in prayer, in a potato field, as the sun sets in the background. In the distance one can perceive the faint outline of a village church steeple, its bells tolling the evening Angelus to call the community to prayer. Looking at this print always makes me want to stop for a moment and pray, wishing that I might be united with these young peasant farmers who had interrupted their field work to pay homage to their Lord.

The attraction to particular religious symbols or religious art will be different, of course, for each of us. But being surrounded by things that touch the heart and lift the spirit can be very helpful in supporting an ongoing prayer life. There will, in the trajectory of one's developing spiritual life, always be times of distraction and dryness; these are dealt with later in the chapter. Nevertheless, using natural God-given gifts such as religious art or uplifting spiritual meditations may strengthen one's commitment to prayer and inspire perseverance in attempting the seemingly impossible gospel mandate to "pray always."

Prayer and Nursing Practice:
A Nurse's Sabbath

There are many ways to approach a discussion of prayer and nursing practice, because our workplaces are so varied in the contemporary profession. We are hospital nurses, clinic nurses, nurse practitioners in offices, home care nurses, long-term care nurses, parish nurses, military nurses, and nurses employed in other disciplines and settings too numerous to name. Within these arenas, we are nurse clinicians, nurse administrators, nurse managers, nurse educators, and nurse researchers. We are told in the gospel of Jesus that when we care for the sick, we care for Him, that, in fact, our nursing becomes our prayer. But are all of our nursing tasks of equal value? Do they all constitute living the gospel message of Jesus?

A tale from the desert fathers reminds us that a great variety of good works are blessed by the Lord: "For scripture says that Abraham was hospitable and God was with him. And David was humble and God was with him. And Elias loved solitary prayer and God was with him. So, do whatever you see your soul desires according to God." (Vincent, 1981, p. 44) I love that desert fathers' story, because it reminds me that there are many options to serving the Lord for us as nurses; there are many prayerful ministries of caring for the sick which reflect the gospel message: "I was ill and you visited me." In order, however, to be sensitive to prayer, to the need for prayer in the nursing workplace, we also need to have some private time, some "Sabbath time," to be alone to talk with and to listen to the Lord.

The Sabbath is an important day for many major religious traditions; it is a time of rest and relaxation from the workweek, but most importantly, it is a time of prayer, both individual prayer and community prayer. Most Christian denominations hold communal worship services each Sunday (or Saturday, for some). For Roman Catholics, Sunday or Saturday evening Mass is a mandate of the Church; and for many Jewish communities, Sabbath temple worship is expected each week. Because of the importance of the concept, theologian Abraham Heschel wrote a book, now a classic, entitled *The Sabbath, Its Meaning for Modern Man*. In the book theologian Heschel wrote: "Six days a week we wrestle with the world, wringing profit from the earth; on the Sabbath we especially care for the seed of eternity planted in the soul. The world has our hands, but our soul belongs to Someone Else." (Heschel, 1979, p. 13)

The problem, of course, is that nurses often do not have a Sabbath in terms of a particular day of the week. Our Sabbath may consist of 8 to 12 hours staffing an intensive care unit or an emergency room; we may be out in the community doing home care visits to those unable to travel because of illness or disability; or we might even be physically at our respective churches, yet involved in such activities as blood pressure screening or health counseling in the role of parish or church nurse. It's true that such nursing ministries can themselves constitute prayerful efforts, yet we truly do need some time and place of Sabbath, apart, for our personal communion with the Lord. How can this be accomplished?

The Sabbath spirituality of Abraham Heschel holds that on the Sabbath we must attempt to avoid the tyranny of things and "try to become attuned to holiness in time." (Heschel, p. 10) I would suggest that because we nurses may not always have one full Sabbath day during a week, although when possible that would surely be desirable, we may, instead, try to create several small Sabbath experiences within the seven-day period. During those mini-Sabbath times, we can embrace Heschel's concept of becoming "attuned to holiness." Our Sabbath experiences might take place on a quiet Sunday evening, a free Wednesday morning, or a Friday afternoon, before a family dinner or weekend activities take over our lives. Communal worship services may need to be worked around our nursing schedules, but this is not always possible. Nurses are consummate improvisors; one thing I am certain of is that if a nurse sets out to make something work, it will work.

What I am suggesting is surely not new; it's the way a number of nurses have created their Sabbath times for many years. In the early days of nursing education, or "training" as we called it back then, students, and sometimes graduate nurses, had only one free afternoon a week and that rarely fell on a Saturday or a Sunday. And yet, as our history documents, nurses throughout the centuries have included a prayerful spirituality as a significant dimension of their nursing practice. The challenge for us, as contemporary nurses, is to continue in the footsteps of those who have gone before us and to continue our commitment to a prayerful and sacred covenant of caring as we carry out our nurse-patient inter-actions in the sophisticated health care milieu of the twenty-first century.

Prayer and Emotions in Nursing: The Lamp Is Heavy

Most spiritual writers consider the concept of one's emotions or feelings as a relevant dimension of prayer. Emotions occurring in or around prayer may be positive, as the example of "feeling" God's presence and love; they may be negative relating to anger at or frustration with God for some perceived offense or unmet need. One can also have feelings of anxiety, fear, or guilt related to our relationship or lack of relationship with the Lord. Jesuit William Barry asserts that if we want to develop a relationship with God we must be willing to share our emotions and feelings as well as our thoughts. (Barry, 1987, p. 47) It has been reported that "the early Christians were not at all afraid of being emotional in prayer"; (Tugwell, 1974, p. 45) and that "when we hold nothing back from God, we eventually come to see that He has been hold-ing nothing back from us." (Billy, 1998, p. 54) Related also to including emotions in prayer are using both intuition, or the right-brain "being" side of our nature; (Oliva, 1994, p. 74) and imagination, which can "open us up to the mystery of God's trans-forming presence within us." (Bergan & Schwan, 1986, p. 10)

The easy part, for me at least, of incorporating emotion into prayer is the use of positive emotions; I delight in "feeling" the joy and the peace and the comfort of the gifts of God and of the pres-ence of God in my life and in the lives of others. It's easy to pray happily and gratefully about those things. It's much harder to talk to the Lord about my pain or my anger or my frustration. It just doesn't seem appropriate to bring up negative thoughts or feelings in prayer. Somehow I think that if I don't talk to God about things that are painful to discuss, maybe He won't know what I'm feel-ing. That is surely a very foolish perception if I really believe, as I say, that God is the center of my life and knows me even better than I know myself.

A nurse friend, who is much wiser than I, shared a good example of using negative emotion in prayer. She was describing the pain of a patient of hers who had been diagnosed with advanced ovarian cancer; she was a young mother with school-age children. The patient confessed that she was very angry with God about her illness and could no longer pray at all. My friend told her gently that she understood why she might feel angry at God, but she advised her, "don't hold it in; you don't have to carry this burden alone. Tell God how angry you are; yell at Him if you want to. God has very strong shoulders. He can take it." My friend's patient told her later that the angry emotional prayer had provided a breakthrough; she could now pray and cry and be angry, yet she had also regained her faith that God was listening to her and loving her, and that He would be with her in whatever she had yet to endure.

When I hear nursing stories like this one, I realize how really heavy a nurse's lamp is some days. As suggested earlier, we can pray for and with our patients; we can listen to them and advise them; we can be present in their times of need. It's almost impossible, however, not to take on some of their pain, which must then be included in our own prayer life, in our own relationship with the Lord. And this is what we often neglect to do in prayer. Think about some recent experience in your hospital, your clinic, your school of nursing, or a patient's home, when you felt deeply a patient, family, or student's personal suffering. Probably you talked about the situation with a close friend or family member— someone who would understand, and care, and share with you a little the burden of suffering you yourself were experiencing. But did you speak about your pain, in prayer, with the Lord?

Personally, I'm sometimes guilty of thinking, if I'm dealing with a very difficult problem, that I'm just too distracted to pray, that I'm so concerned about whatever situation has captured my attention that I just can't be "recollected" or "prayerful" right now.

I tend to think: "I'll pray later, when I'm feeling up to it." Not a good strategy. Later may never come, or if it does, I have carried a heavy emotional burden alone for a long time before I finally get around to laying it at the feet of my Lord and my God and asking for help. He waits for us to bring Him our pain, our distraction, and our dryness just as anxiously as He waits for our love and our adoration. That is the consummate blessing of a prayerful relationship with the Lord.

Distraction and Dryness in Prayer

I have spent a lot of time exploring books on prayer during the past few years; and virtually all of the spiritual writers in the area include a chapter, or at least a portion of a chapter, on the problems of "distraction" and/or "dryness." Peter Kreeft, in his book *Prayer for Beginners* promises that anyone who tries seriously to pray will have distractions: even the saints, he notes "had wandering minds." (Kreeft, 2000, p. 77)

Dryness, or a lack of emotion or feeling in prayer, is often related to the concept of the "dark night of the soul" described by the great Saint John of the Cross. In this context, dryness is seen as "intrinsic" to each person's spiritual journey; (Oliva, 1994, p. 87) and a "good and healthy sign of real interior growth." (Green, 1998, p. 123) The suffering associated with dryness in prayer is also related to the Gospel message of Jesus: "If any want to follow me, let them ... take up their Cross (Matthew 16: 24); and "Unless a grain of wheat falls into the earth and dies, it remains only a grain" (John 12: 24). (Green, 1998, p. 81)

Describing the benefits of distraction in prayer, Mary Clare Vincent, OSB asserts that "distractions are not only inevitable, they are indispensable." (Vincent, 1982, p. 67) Vincent's point is that distractions help us to recognize our own weakness and dependence upon God; they also provide the opportunity to refine our faithfulness to prayer even as we struggle. (Vincent, p. 67) Periodic dryness can be very fruitful because during such times "our prayer is likely to be most unselfish, most God-centered" as we continue to persevere in prayer through such feelings as apathy or emptiness. (Green, 1998, p. 105)

For us, as nurses, I think that the topics of distraction, dryness, and unanswered prayer are particularly difficult, because we are used to achieving our goals; nurses are primarily "do-ers" rather than "be-ers." We have been educated from early nursing courses that assigned tasks must be accomplished and accomplished well; our patients' lives may depend on it. Thus, it is not easy to simply wait; to simply, as asked by the Lord: "Be still and know that I am God." That, however, is precisely what we must do when we experience the kinds of prayer hindrances described above. We must put aside our goal-oriented mentality, surrender our needs and desires to God, and accept that so often His time and His will are not ours. This is the key to faithfulness in developing a prayer life and in developing a relationship with God. This is the faith that will carry us through on the darkest days when we feel lonely and wounded, that will allow us to become ourselves wounded healers.

Preparation for Prayer: Five Steps

I have written about the history of prayer in nursing, the prayer and nurse-patient relationships, the need for prayer in nursing, and the difficulties one might experience such as distraction and dryness in prayer. But how does one begin to pray, or how can one strengthen or improve one's current prayer life? What should one say in prayer? These are questions frequently asked by those who are serious about developing or strengthening a relationship with the Lord.

Another frequently asked question about prayer is "are there techniques or methods of prayer one should use?" I feel ambivalent about addressing the idea of "methods" of prayer because personal prayer may vary greatly depending upon an individual's personality, needs, experience, and religious tradition. One spiritual writer suggests that love is "too simple, too free and too great" for techniques or methods; (Kreeft, 2000, pp. 49–50) another feels that we do need a few methods that "fit us the best" but that we should avoid becoming overburdened by too many techniques of prayer. (Wolff, 1995, p. 38) I personally believe that where one is in the process of developing his or her relationship with the Lord will dictate which, if any, methods will be helpful; the methods used may also change across one's lifetime as life stages and life demands change.

Having said all that, I have to admit that I am still asked by colleagues to identify some steps to take in preparing oneself for a time of prayer. Although I am loathe to interfere with the action of the Holy Spirit, perhaps a few of the practical steps I personally have used might be helpful. *First*, I try to block out some uninterrupted time for prayer; this block of time may be in the morning, the evening, or any time in between, when I think I might be able to escape the telephone, email, or face-to-face interactions with others besides the Lord. He is my best friend, after all, and surely deserves my full attention when we are together. *Second*, I look for a place to pray that will be both quiet and relatively comfortable. While I usually prefer to pray in a chapel or church, I have often found my own room to be a wonderfully peaceful setting for prayer. Some things that help me settle down in this space, after a busy day, are the lighting of a candle and/or playing religious music softly; I also like sitting on the floor or using a small prayer bench to place my body in a prayerful attitude. Weather permitting, the outdoors can also provide a magnificent natural prayer environment; some days I just like to go for a walk with the Lord.

A *third* step to beginning a time of prayer, which I have discussed earlier, might be to open the Bible to a favorite passage; this step helps orient one's mind away from the problems of the day, or perhaps even toward the problems of the day, but in the light of God's love and guidance rather than one's own insights. If I am really worried about something, a passage from one of the psalms of God's protecton is a powerful reminder of the Lord's care, for example: "You know when I sit down and when I rise up...you lay your hand upon me ... behind and before you encircle me and rest your hand upon me" (Psalm 139, v.1; 5); or "God...will not let your foot be moved, he who keeps you will not slumber...the Lord will keep your going out and your coming in" (Psalm 121, v.3; 8).

A *fourth* step in preparation for prayer is to become interiorly quiet before the Lord. This step may be the most difficult in preparing for a time of prayer; at least, it can be for me. I sometimes feel like I have spent the first half or even three quarters of the time I had allotted for prayer trying to clear my mind, to let go of the many "important" thoughts running around in my head, either from the day that has just ended or regarding the day that is about to begin. I have to keep reminding myself that the most "important" thing I can do in prayer is just be present to the Lord; unfortunately, I am a very slow learner.

And then, after the first four steps have been taken, the most important step in beginning to pray is, of course, to listen. Surely it is a good thing to ask that our needs be met, to tell the Lord about our concerns for ourselves and for our loved ones, but the ultimate goal of a developing prayer life is to learn to listen to the Lord. The Holy Spirit's whisperings and His guidance can only be heard in the silence of a quiet soul, in the silence of an undistracted mind, and in the silence of an undivided heart. This focus is what we must attempt to bring to our times of prayer: a mind and a spirit totally focused on the One who is the center of our lives and the source of our strength, and a heart filled with love for Him, who alone can ease the yearning described so poignantly by Augustine: "Our hearts are restless, O Lord, until they rest in Thee."

For those of us who have busy schedules most days of the week, a structured morning prayer can be very helpful in setting a tone for the day. I find it important to attend Mass and pray the morning prayer of the Divine Office each day; that arrangement may not work for others depending upon religious tradition, work schedule, or prayer needs. I do feel, however, that to plan on some time for prayer on arising, even if abbreviated, is both necessary and comforting for those of us who care for the sick (or who teach or supervise those who minister to the ill). It's also very important for developing our relationship with God. Imagine if, in your household, you got up in the morning, showered, dressed, had your coffee or filled a cup to take in the car, and rushed out the front door without even saying "good morning" to the people with whom you live. You may just give your loved ones a quick "good morning" greeting or a hug; the point is that you have done something to make a connection. You have acknowledged, even if briefly, the love that exists between you and the significant others in your life; should it not be the same with the one who is the greatest love of our lives? Why should we as nurses pray? How can we not pray!

We Hold This Treasure

Dear Lord Jesus,
Help us never to forget the "treasure" we hold (2 Cor. 4:7);
The "treasure" which graces our earthen vessels with
Your compassion and Your care.

Bless our earthen vesselness,
that we may be instruments of Your "surpassing
power" (2 Cor. 4:7):

to teach the insecure;
to counsel the confused;
to advise the anxious;
to advocate for the helpless; and
to bring the light of
Your loving Spirit
to those who suffer.

References

Barry, W. A. (1987). *God and you: Prayer as a personal relationship.* New York: Paulist Press.

Bergan, J. and Schwan, M. (1986). *A guide for prayer.* Winona, MN: Saint Mary's Press.

Billy, D. (1998). *Soliloquy prayer: Unfolding our hearts to God.* Liguori, MO: Liguori Publications.

Casey, M. (1996). *Toward God: The ancient wisdom of western prayer.* Liguori, MO: Liguori/Triumph.

(1987). *Collegeville series on books of the bible.* Collegeville, MN: The Liturgical Press.

Dossey, B. M. (2000). *Florence Nightingale: Mystic, visionary, healer.* Springhouse, PA: Springhouse Corporation.

Green, T. H. (1998). *When the well runs dry: Prayer beyond the beginnings.* Notre Dame, IN: Ave Maria Press.

Groeschel, B. J. (1984). *Listening at prayer.* New York: Paulist Press.

Heschel, A. (1979). *The Sabbath: Its meaning for modern man.* New York: Ferrar, Straus and Giroux.

Kreeft, P. (2000). *Prayer for beginners.* San Francisco: Ignatius Press.

Lawrence of the Resurrection. (1973). *The practice of the presence of God.* Mount Vernon, NY: Peter Pauper Press.

Macrae, J. (1995). Nightingale's spiritual philosophy and its significance for modern nursing, *Image* 27 (1), 10-13.

Nightingale, F. (1859). *Notes on nursing: What it is and what it is not.* London: Harrison.

O'Brien, M.E. (2003). *Spirituality in nursing: Standing on holy ground.* Sudbury, MA: Jones and Bartlett Publishers.

Oliva, M. (1994). *Free to pray: Free to love.* Notre Dame, IN: Ave Maria Press.

Tugwell, S. (1974). *Prayer in practice.* Springfield, IL: Templegate Publishers.

Vincent, M.C. (1981). *The life of prayer and the way to God.* Petersham, MA: Saint Bede's Press.

Wolff, P. (1995). *The hungry heart.* Liguori, MO: Triumph Books.

Zyromski, P. (2000). *Pray the bible.* Cincinnati, OH: St. Anthony Messenger Press.

Nursing in the Twenty-First Century:
A Nurse's Prayer for the
Third Millenium

A Nurse's Prayer for the Third Millennium

O Lord, Our God,
the world of this third millennium
struggles with pain and suffering,
the depth of which You, alone, truly know.
Guide us, as nurses, to use our
chosen ministry to alleviate at least
a part of the anxiety, the fear,
the insecurity, the sorrow, and the grief,
with which so many of Your people are burdened.
Mentor us to be ministers of Your love
and Your compassion
as we teach,
as we counsel,
as we advocate,
as we advise,
and as we attempt to bring
Your Blessed Presence to console
the spirits of those who are wounded.
We are gifted to be allowed to serve
as ministers of Your gospel.
Help us to be worthy.

Nurses' Prayers for the Sick

Prayer for a Person Preparing to Enter the Hospital

The Lord is my light and my salvation; whom shall I fear?

PSALM 27:1

Dear Lord,
You know that this is an anxious time for [name],
as [he/she] prepares to enter the hospital.
Hospitals are blessed places where healing and helping
take place; but hospitals are also houses
of the unknown, of things out of our control.
Remind [name], O Lord, that nothing is out of reach
of Your ever present caring and compassion;
that You are, indeed, [his/her] "life's refuge."
Help [name] to be comforted in the fact that [he/she]
does not take this journey alone;
You are always at [his/her] side: guiding, protecting,
supporting, strengthening, and loving.
Bless [name] with courage, strength, and peace that this
hospitalization may provide a time of rest and
restoration; that [he/she] may soon be gifted
with the recovery which is Your gift
and Your grace. Amen.

Prayer before Surgery

When you walk through fire, you shall not be burned.

ISAIAH 43:2

Dear Lord Jesus,
None of us looks forward to surgery; the
anticipation itself may make us feel as if we are
about to "walk through fire"; and yet, surgery is
truly a precious and a healing gift, with which
You have graced our world, O Lord.
For it is sometimes only through this
painful "walk through fire" that our wounded
bodies may be made whole.
Bless the hands of [name]'s surgeon that they may
be instruments of Your healing and Your love.
Bless [name]'s spirit that [he/she] may be strong
and courageous as [he/she] takes on this new
challenge which You place before [him/her].
While [Name] knows that [he/she] is about to
"walk through fire," [he/she] trusts firmly in Your
caring commitment that, as promised in scripture,
[he/she] "shall not be burned." Amen.

Prayer for a Sick Child

People were bringing even infants to him that he might
touch them . . . Jesus...called [the children] . . . and said . . .
the kingdom of God belongs [to them].

LUKE 18:15–17

Dear Lord Jesus,
You treasured children so much that You taught
our hearts should become like theirs if we would enter
the kingdom of heaven; and You would not allow
anyone to keep the children from You.
Be with [name], this beloved child of Yours, now in
[his/her] illness and suffering.
Gather [name] into Your caring arms during [his/her]
time of sickness and grant [him/her] the peace,
and the comfort, and the rest which You alone can give.
Let [name] know how much You love [him/her]
and that You suffer with [him/her] in [his/her] hurting.
Protect, bless, guard, and comfort [name] with the caring
and compassion which You alone can give. Amen.

Prayer for a Person Beginning Life in a Nursing Home

Do not worry about your life, what you will eat, or about
your body and what you will wear.

LUKE 12:22

Dear Father in heaven,
[Name] is about to take a very important step in [his/her]
life journey; it is a transition that can be frightening, and
yet it is a transition that is also most blessed.
For, here, in the nursing home, the cares and worries
of the world are placed literally in Your hands.
Now it is time for [name] to enter into the
contemplative phase of [his/her] life; this is a grace
which was not possible in the midst of the busyness
of [name]'s former life commitments.
[Name]'s new ministry is now only to live in
Your love and Your light and to share these with
those [he/she] meets each day.
Bless [name] and grace [his/her] nursing home ministry
of presence with Your spirit of peace and prayerfulness.
Let [name] be to all [he/she] meets a beacon of
Your love and Your gentleness. Amen.

Prayer for One Who Is Cognitively Impaired

> *Nor height, nor depth . . . will be able to separate us from the love of God in Christ Jesus our Lord.*
>
> ROMANS 8:3

Dear Father in heaven,
You alone, who created us in Your image and likeness,
can understand the illness that has taken away the
beautiful thoughts and feelings with which
[name]'s human spirit was once gifted.
This is a very painful thing for those of us
who love [him/her]. And yet, we know that
You do not reside in [name]'s mind, or even in [his/her]
heart but rather in the depths of [name]'s soul;
in a place where no illness which ravages the human
body, no disease which destroys the human mind,
can ever reach.
Neither the heights of wisdom nor the depths of confusion can "separate" [name] from the love of Your Divine
Son. Bless [name] in the gentle mist of confusion which
has become [his/her] earthly home. And take [name], one
day, to [his/her] heavenly home where, with the angels
and saints, [he/she] will again be able to praise Your
glory with the joy and the understanding that You alone
can give. Amen.

Prayer for an Unconscious Person

> *O Lord, you have searched me and known me . . . you dis-*
> *cern my thoughts from far away.*

PSALM 139:1–2

Gentle Lord,
You know that [name] is no longer able to pray for
[him/herself]. We do not know where [his/her] spirit
now rests, but we trust that it is held tenderly in Your
beloved hands.
[Name's] ability to speak words of prayer are not important to You, Lord God of life, for you "have probed"
[him/her] and "You know" [him/her] both from near and
"from afar." [He/she] is Your beloved child and [his/her]
name is written in the palm of Your hand.
Bless [name] with Your compassionate care and hold
[him/her] close to Your loving heart during this time
of fragility and weakness.
Let [name] hear Your voice in the stillness and silence of
[his/her] immortal soul. Amen.

Prayer for Healing

*I know the plans I have for you, says the Lord, plans for
your welfare, and not for harm!*

JEREMIAH 29:11

Dear Father in heaven,
We pray now for healing for [name]. We pray that
[he/she] will be healed, in body and in spirit, from this
illness which has invaded [his/her] life. We pray for this
physical healing, Dear Lord, but only if it is Your
blessed will.
You alone know what is needed for [name]'s life,
for as taught by the prophet Jeremiah,
You "know well the plans"
You have in mind for [name]; "plans for [his/her]
welfare, not for [his/her] woe."
Thus, as we beg this healing, of [name]'s body or spirit, we
ask also "let us pray" in the precious words of Your Son,
Our Lord Jesus: "If it be possible let the chalice pass"
from [name], yet not [his/her] will but Thine be done.
Amen.

Prayer for Strength in Suffering

> *My help comes from the Lord, who made heaven and earth.*
>
> PSALM 121:1

Dearest Lord,
It's not easy for [name] to pray in the midst of
[his/her] suffering; sometimes the pain is overwhelming.
We beg You to become [name's] strength and help
[him/her] in the midst of these difficult days.
Wrap [him/her] in Your loving arms and cradle [his/her]
suffering soul in a blanket of Your tender care.
Breathe Your Blessed strength into [name's] spirit, that
[he/she] may gain the courage to accept, the courage to
endure, and, at times, even the courage to weep.
Make of [name's] suffering a crucible within which
Your grace and Your beauty will shine forth to all
[he/she] meets, O God of miracles and wonders. Amen.

Prayer for Acceptance of God's Will

> *Can I not do with you . . . as this potter has done? says the Lord. Just like the clay in the potter's hand, so are you in my hand.*

> JEREMIAH 18:6

Dear Father in heaven,
You asked the prophet Jeremiah if You could
do with him "as the potter has done." To remold him in
the image You would have him become. This is what
You are asking of [name].
But this is not an easy thing for [him/her] to accept,
Dear Lord: to have [his/her] life plans dismantled,
disorganized, or even destroyed,
that [he/she] may be remolded as Your will allows.
Bless [name] with Your courage, with Your strength,
and with Your peace, in the midst of this time of
challenge and suffering.
Help [name] to accept a plan that is not [his/hers].
Be to [him/her] a refuge, where [he/she] might
seek peaceful shelter until the storm has passed. Amen.

Prayer of Thanksgiving for Recovery from Illness

> *For now the winter is past, the rain is over and gone.*
>
> THE SONG OF SONGS 2:11

Dear Lord Jesus,
Thank you for the blessing of [name]'s recovery from
[his/her]illness. Let [him/her] rejoice in this precious
springtime of Your love, for at last "the winter is past"
and the "rains are over and gone."
Bless [name] with the grace of gratitude for the gift of
health and the gift of strength.
Guide [him/her] to use this treasure to share Your love
and Your compassion in the ministry of Your gospel
message to all [he/she] meets.
We praise You, O Lord, for Your care;
we praise You, O Lord, for Your compassion;
we praise You, O God of life and resurrection,
for Your tender love and merciful heart. Amen.

Prayer for One Who Is Terminally Ill

Unless a grain of wheat falls into the earth and dies, it remains just a single grain; but if it dies, it bears much fruit.

JOHN 12:24

Dear Lord Jesus,
You taught that the "grain of wheat must fall
to the ground and die" in order to bear fruit;
You, who came to know so intimately the lesson of
that fallen "grain"! This is now the message
which [name] has heard!
Strengthen [him/her] with the courage which You
alone can give.
The "grain" of [name]'s earthly life is preparing
to fall to the ground that [his/her] heart's legacy
may bear fruit for generations to come.
Let [name]'s falling be as gentle as an autumn leaf
drifting slowly, rhythmically, tenderly, downward
as it blankets the chilled earth with a splendid quilt of
orange and red.
Grace the world with the precious coverlet of [name]'s
life and love, that [his/her] spirit may
endure forever. Amen.

Prayer for a Person Entering a Hospice

Do not fear those who kill the body but cannot kill the soul.

MATTHEW 10:28

Dear Lord Jesus,
[Name], your beloved [son/daughter], is about to
embark on [his/her] final journey to the blessed place
which you promised to prepare for all of us.
The enemy of illness has ravaged the earthly body of
[name] but [his/her] soul grows stronger and more beautiful each day.
As Saint Paul taught so many centuries ago, "even
though our outer nature is wasting away, our inner
nature is being renewed day by day" (2 Corinthians 4:16).
"For this," Paul added, "slight momentary affliction
is preparing for us for an eternal weight of glory
beyond all measure" (17).
Help [name] in this time of [his/her] life transition,
to look, with Paul, "not what can be seen but
what cannot be seen; for what can be seen is temporary,
but what cannot be seen is eternal" (18). Amen.

Prayer for Discontinuing Life Support

For everything there is a season . . . a time to be born and a time to die.

ECCLIASTES 3:1–2

Dear Father in heaven,
We are about to give our dear [name] into Your
tender and loving care.
You know how hard it is for us to let go!
We have loved [name] in health and in illness;
we have loved [name] in joy and sorrow;
we have loved [name] in strength and suffering.
Our earthly world will never be the same without
[name]. But now it is time for [name]'s heavenly
reward; now it is time for us to surrender
[him/her] into Your loving arms.
Bring [name] into the company of the angels and
saints; let [him/her] live forever in Your
tender care, and let [name]'s memory live
each day in the hearts of those who loved [him/her].
Amen.

Prayer for One Experiencing Grief or Loss

> *Blessed are those who mourn, for they will be comforted.*
>
> MATTHEW 5:4

Dear Father,
You know that [name] is grieving deeply
right now. We know that you have promised comfort
to those who mourn, but sometimes it seems a long
time in coming.
Grant [name] peace and patience during this
time of loss and grieving.
Bless [him/her] with Your loving care and compassion
that [he/she] may face each day supported by the tender
awareness of Your presence and Your love.
Help [name] to know that [he/she] is never
alone in [his/her] grieving but is always accompanied by
Your Blessed Spirit of wisdom and understanding.
Grace [name] with healing. Amen.

Prayer in Bereavement

I am the resurrection and the life. Those who believe in me,
even though they die, will live and everyone who lives and
believes in me will never die.

JOHN 11:25–26

Dearest Lord Jesus,
[Name] has lost [his/her] beloved [spouse/parent/child];
no words can ease the pain of this terrible suffering.
[Name]'s only true comfort can come from You
alone, Lord God of life, and death,
who promised in Your own blessed words:
"I am the resurrection and the life;
whoever believes in me, even if he dies,
will live and whoever lives and
believes in me will never die."
Bless [name] with Your tender care and
comfort and help [him/her] to remember
Your promise; that [his/her] beloved [name] is not dead,
but lives in glory in Your heavenly kingdom,
where one day [they] will be reunited
among the company of the blessed. Amen.

A Nurse's Psalm of Reverence for Life

A Nurse's Psalm of Reverence for Life

Oh, Lord our God, I praise you
for the gift of life.
When I see a newborn infant, the
work of your hands;
A mother's love, the tenderness
of your care.

Who are we that you bless us
with the sacredness of life;
that you create us to serve
each other with caring
and compassion.

For the chronically ill, who find in
their infirmities, the power
of your strength, I praise you O Lord.

For the mentally challenged, who engage
their lives with bravery and gentleness,
I praise you O Lord.

For the physically handicapped, who clothe
their disabilities with dignity and grace,
I praise you O Lord.

For sick children, who embrace their
illnesses with courage and
simplicity, I praise you O Lord.

For frail elders, who boldly refuse
to "go gently" into the night,
I praise you O Lord.

For loving families, who tenderly
support disabled members,
I praise you O Lord.

For loyal friends, who faithfully
attend to the needs of ill comrades,
I praise you O Lord.

For the blessing, and the holiness
and the giftedness of all human life,
I praise and thank you
O Lord.

A Nurse's Way of the Cross

Nurses, in the course of their profession, may experience their own unique way of the Cross, through encountering and embracing their patients' sufferings. These observations and inter-actions can be included in a nurse's prayer life through associating his or her patients' agonies with those of Our Blessed Lord in meditations and prayers that constitute a "Nurse's Way of the Cross."

1. Jesus Is Condemned To Die.

He's a fine young man, a boy really, only 16 when the symptoms first start: the headaches, the dizziness, and the nausea. Not so bad, at first; probably too many hours on the new computer he thinks, or maybe just worry about those upcoming SATs. But then one morning he can't get out of bed and the round of testing begins, and the surgery. An invasive glioblastoma, the neurosur-geon said; we couldn't get it all. He is condemned to die, this innocent, whose only crime was choosing to embrace his teenage life.

> Dear Lord Jesus, who in Your own innocence, was con-demned to die for choosing to embrace our fragile world, help my patients to embrace their physical condemnations. I get angry sometimes; it seems so unfair. I can't under-stand; I don't ask to. Only grant me the grace to cross over; to stand as Your loving presence with those condemned to death from illness or disease.

2. Jesus Takes Up His Cross.

"The breast cancer has spread to the lymph nodes," they tell the young mother. There's a husband and two toddlers to think of; "we'll begin an aggressive program of treatment" the oncology team advises. "We can't save your hair, not with this much chemotherapy," they admit, but "don't worry, the wigs they make these days are pretty good." "Mommy, Mommy, pick me up," the little ones cry in unison. "Mommy loves you so much," she replies, "but right now Mommy is sick. She has to rest. But don't ever forget: Mommy loves you!"

> Blessed Lord Jesus, you took up such a heavy Cross for us. Help me to accept the crosses that sickness and disability impose. Taking up a cross is a fearful task but You, Dear Lord, blessed the action with Your love and compassion. Teach me to help my patients look to You for courage and strength as they struggle to take up their personal crosses.

3. Jesus Falls for the First Time.

Everything seems to be going well with the new therapeutic regimen. The brittle juvenile onset diabetes that has dominated his life for so many years is under control. The disease is a cross but it's become manageable, or so the young teacher thinks. All he wants is to enjoy the end of school party with his class of boisterous eighth graders. They don't understand his need for a delicate balance of exercise, diet, and medication. He wakes up that evening in the medical ICU; the hurt to his body is modest, the hurt to his spirit grievous.

> Dearest Jesus, it's really hard to fall when you think that the path before you will be smooth. It hurts not only the body but also the heart. Help me to be there to catch my patients when they fall; help me especially to catch their spirits that I might lift them up to you.

4. Jesus Meets His Sorrowful Mother.

She's a small woman, with dark hair, no grey yet or at least she hides it well, and a kind and gentle smile; only her eyes reveal the terrible sadness in her heart. "This is my Mom" the young cancer patient says proudly. He has something called stage IV rhabdomyosarcoma; it's too horrible a label for a 21 year old, and he's in the advanced stages of the disease. The mother's courage is overwhelming. In his room she teases, cajoles, supports, and loves; she is his mother. In the hallway she dissolves into heart-wrenching sobs; she is his mother.

> Blessed Lord, Your own beloved mother's heart was pierced
> by a cruel sword. Help me to minister to the mothers and
> fathers of my young patients. Teach me to touch their pain
> with gentleness, so that I may stand with them as a caring
> companion on their journeys of suffering. Help me, also, to
> be myself a "mother" to those for whom I care.

5. Simon of Cyrene Helps Jesus Carry His Cross.

Paul, the young unit clerk on the childrens' oncology ward is bald; I mean really bald, like the proverbial "billiard ball." I asked the staff about it. "Is he a chemo patient himself?" I wondered, or "Is shaving off all one's hair some kind of contemporary statement?" "Oh, it's definitely a statement," the nursing staff replied. "You see, Paul knows how hard it is for the children on chemotherapy to lose their hair; it's especially tough on the teens. So Paul decided to shave off his own hair so that the children won't feel alone. He did it as a sign of support." Amazing! this dear young Paul "of Cyrene."

> Blessed Lord Jesus, the weight of your heavy Cross was
> lightened by the young, strong arms of Simon. Teach me,
> as a nurse, to use my arms and my heart to lighten the
> painful suffering of those I care for. Teach me to have the
> courage of Simon in the practice of my nursing.

6. Veronica Wipes the Face of Jesus.

They brought him into the ER on the rescue squad gurney; it took two paramedics to hold him down. He was fighting the IVs and the oxygen just as he'd always had to fight for his life. That's the way it is living on the mean city streets. When he relaxed a little, a nurse tenderly washed the blood and grit from his eyes and face. "God bless you," he breathed softly through bruised and swollen lips. And God did.

> My dearest Lord, you know about struggling for life. You experienced human cruelty in the most devastating way; you were betrayed by those you came to save. We nurses have the precious gift of being able to comfort our patients as Veronica comforted you in your time of suffering. Teach me to honor and reverence the gift.

7. Jesus Falls for the Second Time.

This time he was "sure he could do it," the ragged, trembling ER patient tells his nurse. Alcohol has ruled his life for so very long. "No more," he had decided, "no more!" Now his eyes reflect the pain and the shame of a resolve shattered and broken. The weight of his addiction is so heavy. He has fallen once again; "yes, it happened before," he admits. But, he desperately struggles to rise again and regain his fragile foothold on life.

> My Dear Lord Jesus, in your blessed humanity, you chose to experience the pain of a heavy Cross, and to embrace the shame of falling beneath its weight. Teach me to accept my own human weaknesses; and teach me never to judge the weaknesses of my patients when they fall.

8. Jesus Comforts the Women of Jerusalem.

His wife and his mother and his sister were all in the room; they looked heartbroken. "Don't be so grim," he teased them with a twinkle in his eye. "I can beat this thing; that tumor's probably been growing for years. I've still got lots of time to get in your hair; you can't get rid of me yet!" He tried to sound gruff but his eyes were filled with love and care for his dear ones and their pain.

> My Beloved Lord, you knew what lay ahead; you knew
> about the suffering and you knew about the shame. Yet, in
> your own terrible pain, you reached out and comforted the
> women who loved you. Help my patients to have the
> strength and the courage to comfort their loved ones; help
> me to lift them up to you in their sorrow that they also may
> be comforted.

9. Jesus Falls for the Third Time.

This one was supposed to be the winner. Twice before a donated kidney had become available, but the match just wasn't there. This time it was, the surgeon said: "Well, maybe not perfect but good enough." And for a while the "good enough" seemed to hold. But then the rejection symptoms began; mild at first, but soon beyond all help. Despite the nephrology team's "full court press," she has to return to dialysis. It's a crushing fall.

> My Lord Jesus, when you experienced that third painful fall
> it must have been devastating. Did you wonder if you could
> rise again and complete the awful journey? Help me to
> reach out to my patients when they fall. Help me to help
> them stand and embrace their journey of living.

10. Jesus Is Stripped of His Garments.

They rushed him into the burn unit in the middle of the night. The fire had incinerated his small frame house in minutes; it stripped off 70 percent of his skin in the process. The pain was unbearable; it couldn't get much worse. He hadn't the strength to moan but his eyes told the tale. We did what we could.

> Dear Lord Jesus, it's so hard to see patients hurting so much, especially when an illness or accident strips them of their human dignity. Help me to remember to always reverence the sacredness of human life.

11. Jesus Is Nailed to the Cross.

This was the first time she would be attached to the hemodialysis machine. She had known it was coming; there was a history of polycystic kidneys. It was the loss of control that seemed the worst part. To be forced to sit, unmoving, while all of her blood is circulating through a monstrous machine. "I feel like I'm about to be nailed to a cross," she sighed.

> Blessed Lord Jesus, it's so very hard to lose control; You know. Teach me to be gentle with my patients in their frustration; teach me to help them bear their losses with grace and with dignity.

12. Jesus Dies on the Cross.

She was only 42 years old but had been on the ventilator for almost three weeks now. The battle with ALS (amyotrophic lateral sclerosis) was long and tortuous; she was more than ready, but the family hadn't been willing to let go. Finally, they said, "Enough, we can't watch her suffer anymore." Her family surrounded the bed; her physician was there, as were the primary care nurse, the hospital chaplain, and a young med student who had grown to love her. They "pulled the plug," but tenderly and with great sadness. They experienced the blessing of praying her into eternal life.

> My dearest Jesus, you knew human death intimately; you who chose to experience the passage in its fullness because you loved so deeply. It's a frightening thing; this letting go of everyone and everything we know. But you taught us to know your Father in heaven. Help me to midwife my patients into His loving presence in eternity.

13. Jesus Is Taken Down from the Cross.

He was a junior student nurse doing his first "clinical" when he pulled the "short straw." We need help with postmortem care they told him. He had cared for the patient just yesterday. Sweet little Mrs. O'Reilly was a fragile 93 year old; she had just succumbed to her most recent stroke. As the student gently washed the body of his patient, he thought: "This is someone's mother; this is someone's wife, this is someone's friend." This is Jesus.

> Blessed Lord Jesus, teach me to see you in each patient I care for. It's hard to lose those who have touched our spirits. Help me to remember that they are now with you; that they are not lost to us, and that their memory and all they shared in life will live on in the hearts of those who loved them.

14. Jesus Is Placed in the Tomb.

I didn't want to go to the funeral. He was so young, only 26 years old. I had grown to love him during those last months of the toxoplasmosis battle; I wanted to remember him as strong and vital; the way he was when first we met. It was just too soon for a funeral. But he had asked for a celebration of his life. So, celebrate we did, through the tears and the laughter and the terrible ache that squeezed your heart like a tight steel band. It was just too soon!

> You understand, dearest Lord Jesus. You were only 33 years old and it seemed just too soon for you also. But You, the Divine Son, knew that Your Father's time is not our time. And you embraced the tomb that we might celebrate your life forever. Teach us to treasure the magnificent gift that your death and entombment was for us: Jesus of Nazareth, who died and rose and became for all humanity, Jesus, the Christ.

15. Jesus Is Risen from the Dead.

The Mass of Christian Burial is over. The service had been poignant and healing; the sympathy of family and friends had been genuine and loving. But now the parents must go home, alone, to enter the barren house that once echoed with childhood laughter. The tomb is empty; how can they bear the loss? They hold each other gently and remember the words their pastor had quoted so tenderly from scripture: "I am the resurrection and the life; whoever believes in me even if he dies, will live; and everyone who lives and believes in me will never die" (John 11:25). Their precious child now lives with the Lord; this is their consolation and their strength.

Dear Risen Lord Jesus, who promised life to all who
believe in you, comfort those who mourn. Ease the grievous loss of loved ones with the gift of hope in a promise of
eternal salvation. Grant the bereaved the blessing of your
tender love in their time of sorrow and lead them, finally, to
Your Sacred Heart, where alone they may find solace and
peace.

INDEX

Note: Scripture passages appear in boldface type.